no newer edition
EA/7/2012

DATE DUE

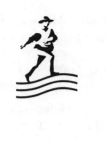

THE
ARTHRITIS
Action
Program

An Integrated Plan of Traditional and Complementary Therapies

A HARVARD MEDICAL SCHOOL BOOK

Michael E. Weinblatt, M.D.

Simon & Schuster

New York London Toronto Sydney Singapore

SIMON & SCHUSTER
Rockefeller Center
1230 Avenue of the Americas
New York, NY 10020

Copyright © 2000 by the President and Fellows of Harvard College

All rights reserved, including the right of reproduction in whole
or in part in any form.

SIMON & SCHUSTER and colophon are registered trademarks
of Simon & Schuster, Inc.

Designed by Stratford Publishing Services, Inc.

Manufactured in the United States of America

1   3   5   7   9   10   8   6   4   2

Library of Congress Cataloging-in-Publication Data
Weinblatt, Michael E.
The Arthritis action program : an integrated plan of traditional and
complementary therapies / Michael E. Weinblatt.
p. cm.
"A Harvard Medical School book."
Includes bibliographical references and index.
1. Arthritis.   2. Arthritis—Alternative treatment.   I. Title.
RC933.W43 2000
616.7'2206—dc21
00-057340
ISBN 0-684-86802-4

Acknowledgments

THIS BOOK reflects a team approach to treating arthritis; in many ways it was a team effort to write, as well. My thanks, first of all, to Ann MacDonald, the writer, who shaped my thoughts and ideas into a coherent and lucid whole. She was a pleasure to work with. I am also grateful to my colleagues at Brigham and Women's Hospital who shared their expertise: Cynthia C. George, M.B.A., P.T. C.H.T., and Marie Weafer-Hodgins, P.T., who provided detailed information about physical and occupational therapy; and Jeffrey N. Katz, M.D., and Agnes Lee Maier, for reviewing drafts of the manuscript and making many helpful suggestions for improving it.

I would also like to thank Walter Willett, M.D., at the Harvard School of Public Health for his contributions to the nutrition sections of this book. Warmest thanks to Glenda Gaines, Jim Moody, and Kelley Sheahan of the American College of Rheumatology, who provided access to experts on various topics, and to the staff of the Arthritis Foundation, who provided helpful background information and patient educational materials.

Finally, I would like to thank my editor at Simon & Schuster, Roslyn Siegel, for her suggestions and advice along the way; assistant editor Andrea Au, for shepherding the manuscript through the publications process; Rose Ann Ferrick and Isolde C. Sauer, for copy editing; Anthony L. Komaroff, M.D., editor in chief of Harvard Health Publications, who saw a need for this book; Victoria Reeders, M.D., publications director of HHP, who helped turn it from vision into reality; and their assistants who expedited the process, notably Matthew Brim and Cara Gibilisco.

For my wife, BARBARA

And for my patients, who are
a continual source of inspiration

Contents

THE ARTHRITIS
Action Program

Introduction

ONE OF the reasons I became a rheumatologist was the wonderful people I met who had developed arthritis and other types of rheumatic diseases. In my twenty-two years of practice, it has been a pleasure to get to know them, and a privilege to treat them.

They are the inspiration for this book.

The information presented in these pages has also been shaped by my professional experiences. As a physician at Brigham and Women's Hospital, I see patients regularly and conduct research into new therapies, particularly those for rheumatoid arthritis. As a professor of medicine at Harvard Medical School, I help to train the next generation of physicians. And as a member (and now president) of the American College of Rheumatology, I work with colleagues from around the country to evaluate the latest research and develop new guidelines for treatment. In all these endeavors I am constantly reminded of how far we have come in solving the puzzle of arthritis—and how much further we need to go.

In the past five years we have made enormous strides in understanding what causes arthritis, how to delay or at least slow its progression, and how to treat it. New medications such as the COX-2 inhibitors and biological response modifiers have expanded the options we can provide to our patients. This has been an enormously exciting time for research.

But we have faced new challenges as well. Managed care is reshaping medicine and sometimes curtails the number of options we can offer patients. The explosive growth of complementary therapies has resulted in more questions than answers. And the Internet is quickly emerging as a significant new force in health care, with the potential to empower—or overpower—us with information.

If you are someone who has arthritis or you are worried that you may develop it, this book should help you make more informed decisions. The recommendations contained in the following pages are based not only on my own experience, but that of my colleagues in the American College of Rheumatology, Harvard Medical

School, and Brigham and Women's Hospital.

Rheumatology requires a team-oriented approach, and this book reflects that philosophy. In the pages that follow you will find detailed information about diet and exercise, medication strategies, physical and occupational therapy, surgical options, and complementary therapies. You'll also find tips on health insurance coverage and cost of treatments, since these factors should be taken into consideration when making decisions.

I hope that you find this helpful. There is as yet no cure for arthritis, but there are plenty of reasons to remain hopeful and optimistic.

MICHAEL E. WEINBLATT, M.D.
Co-director of Clinical Rheumatology,
    Brigham and Women's Hospital
Professor of Medicine, Harvard Medical School

CHAPTER 1

Arthritis: You Can Do Something About It

I've started to have aches and pains in the morning, just like my mother used to. Does that mean I'm developing arthritis too?

I've read about something called "super aspirins." How can I get them?

What do you think about shark cartilage? My colleague said it can prevent arthritis. Does it really work?

Is there a cure for arthritis?

I ANSWER questions like this every time I meet with patients. Small wonder. Arthritis is incredibly common, affecting about one out of six people in this country. Yet few people think about this disease until they develop those first aches and pains and wonder: Could this be it? Now what?

Perhaps you have asked yourself these questions. And if you are like most people, your understanding of arthritis is based on what your parents or grandparents experienced. That can be depressing. Arthritis is a word that brings to mind many images, most of them negative: age, infirmity, limited mobility, pain.

It doesn't have to be that way. This book is intended to explain, in plain English, what arthritis is, how you can protect your joints (even before you feel those first aches and pains), and what you can do if you develop the disease. The information and recommendations included in this book are based not only on my own experience, but that of other healthcare providers at Harvard Medical School and Brigham and Women's Hospital. We work in teams to provide patient care, so this book reflects a team approach, one that involves the perspective of physicians, nurses, surgeons, physical and occupational therapists, pharmacists, and experts in complementary medicine.

Your grandmother may have taken some aspirin and then taken to her chair when her joints "acted up," but you have many more options to choose from. For starters, we'll encourage you to get out of that chair and start moving, with advice about exercises that are safe for your joints and good for your heart, lungs, and muscles. When the pain seems overwhelming, physical and occupational therapy may offer you the relief and confidence you need to keep moving. Finally, we'll provide information about simple steps you can take to protect your joints by choosing the right footwear, using joint supports when necessary, and learning to "listen" to your joints and the distress signals they sometimes send.

This book will also tell you about some truly exciting new treatments for arthritis. There is much to share. In the past few years a number of new medications have been approved for the treatment of arthritis, including the COX-2 inhibitors, marketed under the brand names *Celebrex* and *Vioxx*. Even more exciting are biological response modifiers such as *Enbrel* and *Remicade*, which appear to slow the progress of some types of arthritis. Meanwhile, we have learned more about the advantages and disadvantages of older medications as well as how to combine some of them for better effect.

Because arthritis is a condition that affects people on so many levels—physically, emotionally, and spiritually—we also have included a section on complementary medicine. For the most part we view these techniques as complements rather than alternatives to conventional therapy. This section will cover complementary medicines ranging from herbal supplements to acupuncture to nutritional supplements. The topics covered are based on actual questions patients have asked me and my colleagues over the years. We will discuss not only those complementary therapies that appear to work, but also those that are still under investigation.

If this sounds overwhelming, don't worry. At the end of the book, after explaining various options in detail, there is a section about how some people have woven the various strands into their own individual arthritis programs. We'll provide suggested programs for individuals ranging from those with a mild form of arthritis to those with a more advanced form of the disease. Discuss them with your own healthcare provider to devise a program that is right for you.

Early Diagnosis and Empowerment

Not only will this book explain what is currently known about arthritis and its treatment, but it will also provide the tools you need to evaluate new arthritis management strategies as they become available.

It is my hope to make you both an optimist and a skeptic. An optimist because the outlook for people with arthritis has changed dramatically in the past few years. Arthritis was once considered an inevitable part of growing older, as much a part of aging as gray hair, and many people think that once you develop arthritis, there is not much you can do except take medication to relieve the pain. Not so. In the past decade we have come to understand better the underlying disease process in arthritis. There are now ways to delay the development of arthritis or at least minimize its effects. There is now more reason for hope than ever before. For the first time even the most conservative doctors and researchers are starting to use the word "breakthrough" when talking about arthritis treatment.

Although we still have a lot to learn, this much is certain: The earlier you are diagnosed and take action to minimize the effects of this disease, the better your chances of maintaining your health and your mobility.

But along with the hope comes hype. Health coverage in the media has increased in quantity but not always in quality. Pharmaceutical advertisements can alert you to new treatments but may not always communicate risks as well as benefits. And the Internet is exploding with medical information, but not all of it is from reliable sources. Many of my patients tell me they are overwhelmed with all the information out there, which can be confusing and contradictory.

So this book will also help you become a skeptic. You will learn to differentiate fact from fallacy, hope from hype. You'll learn how your healthcare provider makes a diagnosis, why he or she recommends a certain treatment, and how to distinguish those treatments that have been proven to work from those that are still under evaluation.

This book aims to empower you as much as inform you so that you will know more about the disease and how to decide among treatment options. It does not endorse any one treatment over another. Rather, it seeks to give you the tools you need to make informed decisions.

A Resource As Well As a Reference

This book is intended to be more than a reference: It should also be your resource as you put together your own arthritis action plan.

We have included lists of questions for your healthcare provider, symptom and medication tracking charts, as well as questions to ask yourself as you consider switching to a new treatment. Please feel free to duplicate any of the tables and charts that have been included.

To make sure you have the most up-to-date information possible, we have also established a website for you to consult periodically. This will enable us to provide you with information about new treatments, complementary medicines, and other arthritis management strategies as they become available. The address is www.health.harvard.edu.

CHAPTER 2

Why Good Joints Go Bad

I used to be an athlete in college. Now I have trouble doing yard work.

I never had to ask for help opening a jar. Now I have to ask my husband to open every new jar we buy in the grocery store.

I get stiff just sitting in a chair or in the car. I feel tired and listless.

Is this arthritis? Why has this happened to me?

CHANCES ARE you seldom think about your joints. Even the most health-conscious of us tend to be more concerned about our risk of heart disease or cancer. Few of us even think about arthritis until we start to feel those first aches and pains and wonder: Is this arthritis? Or just a sign that I'm getting older?

Joints are remarkably functional and resilient, which is why it is so easy to forget all about them until something goes wrong. But if you are truly going to take charge of your health, you need to learn more about what's going on under the surface of your skin.

In this chapter we hope to make you more aware of your joints—how they function when they're healthy and how they become damaged in arthritis. That will make it easier to understand the protection and treatment strategies we'll describe in later chapters.

What Is Arthritis?

Arthritis is the medical term for more than one hundred diseases and disorders that cause joints to become damaged or inflamed, resulting in pain and stiffness. The term is derived from two Greek words: *arthron* (joint) and *itis* (inflammation). Some forms of the disease may affect muscles and connective tissues in the body such as skin.

About 42.7 million Americans, one out of every six, have some type of arthritis. The number is expected to increase in the years ahead as the baby boom generation ages and the U.S. population in general becomes older. By the year 2020, 60 million people are expected to be suffering from arthritis.

The most common type of arthritis is *osteoarthritis,* which afflicts about 21 million Americans. In this form of the disease, bones and cartilage deteriorate, partially as a result of the natural process of aging; pain and stiffness result.

One of the most debilitating forms of arthritis is *rheumatoid arthritis,* which affects some 2 million people in the United States. Rheumatoid arthritis may begin when the bones and joints are still healthy. For reasons that remain unclear, the immune system begins attacking joints; the disease then wreaks further havoc as it progresses.

There are many more types of arthritis as well as conditions with similar symptoms. The chapters that follow will provide more information about the major types and how to differentiate a transient ache from the more persistent pain of arthritis.

Major Types of Arthritis

Osteoarthritis	Infectious arthritis
Inflammatory arthritis	Lyme disease
Rheumatoid arthritis	Other rheumatic diseases
Ankylosing spondylitis	Gout
Juvenile arthritis	
Polymyalgia rheumatica	
Psoriatic arthritis	
Reactive arthritis	
Seronegative arthritis	

Related conditions with symptoms resembling arthritis:

Bursitis	Fibromyalgia
Carpal tunnel syndrome	Tendinitis

What Are the Symptoms of Arthritis?

Although each type of arthritis has its own array of symptoms, the following are the most common:

- Difficulty in performing usual daily tasks such as climbing stairs and opening doors
- Fatigue
- Pain in joints
- Stiffness and loss of motion
- Swelling around the joints

All these symptoms may also apply to other conditions. For that reason it is important to start tracking any symptoms as soon as they begin to bother you. If they persist or do not respond to over-the-counter remedies such as aspirin or *Tylenol,* consult a healthcare provider who can help determine whether you are suffering from arthritis or another condition such as bursitis or tendinitis. (Chapter 4 includes more information on the type of healthcare provider to consult and the questions to ask.)

How Joints Function Normally

There are 206 bones in the human body. Each of them comes together at a juncture known as the *joint.* Both bones and joints are essential to your well-being.

Bones are often thought of as stiff and lifeless, an image that probably has to do with their often being depicted in pictures of skeletons. In fact, bones thrive with activity underneath their hard surface. Arteries running throughout bone carry blood and nutrients. Bone marrow, a spongy area inside the bone cavity, produces a variety of blood cells, including those involved in the immune system's response to any perceived threat.

Joints come in various shapes and types. *Fixed joints* do not move and are connected to one another by fibrous tissue. The bones of the skull come together as a fixed joint. *Hinge joints* allow simple movements such as bending or straightening up. *Pivot joints* enable the rotation of a part of the body, such as turning your head. *Ellipsoidal joints* allow all sorts of movement—up, down, and side to side; the wrist joint is a good example. *Ball-and-socket joints*, such as those found in shoulders and hips, allow the broadest range of motion.

Joints may not be the sexiest parts of the body, but they are among the most useful. Joints enable you to walk in the park, throw a baseball to your child, type emails to friends and colleagues, and swim in the pool at the end of a long day. Without joints, our world would be stiff and constricted.

Mobile joints such as knees and shoulders handle a lot of wear and tear each day. Take a stroll down the street, and you place three times your weight on each foot. Walk a mile, and by some estimates you have placed 63 tons of accumulated pressure on your feet. If you jog or run, you place even greater pressure on your joints.

Fortunately, joints are designed to be remarkably resilient. The ends of most bones are covered with cartilage, a tough spongy material that cushions bones against impact when you walk or sit or reach for something. To add extra protection, the entire joint area is covered by a tissue known as the synovial membrane; it produces a slippery substance known as synovial fluid that lubricates the joint. Outside the membrane, ligaments connect bones to each other, keeping bones in proper alignment. Muscles and tendons help keep joints stable and also provide the strength to move various body parts.

Although cartilage was once regarded as the primary protection for our joints—and it is often referred to as a "shock absorber"— that view has changed. We've come to realize that primary protection is provided by the entire joint structure: bone alignment, muscles, tendons, ligaments, and joint capsule. This enables us to "brace" ourselves as we move, helping us withstand stresses during the day. (And if you have ever stepped off the curb by mistake, jolting yourself, you'll have a sense of what can happen if your muscles and other joint structures aren't braced for a particular movement.) In the new view, cartilage is important, but it provides only secondary shock absorption.

Arthritis develops when joints are damaged in some way. Although the exact location and mechanism of injury varies, depending on the type of arthritis, two major factors appear to be involved: repeated stress on joints over time and biological changes that make joints more susceptible to injury. In that respect, arthritis is similar to many other serious diseases, such as heart disease and cancer, that develop because of a complex interplay of heredity, biology, and environmental factors.

What Goes Wrong in Osteoarthritis

As we age, the cartilage that covers the end of bones begins to wear away. In some people the erosion process is more pronounced. While we don't know what causes cartilage to erode in the first place, we do know a lot about what happens once the process is set in motion.

Cartilage is a resilient, rubbery tissue that covers the ends of bones. There are three main types of cartilage: elastic cartilage (such as that found in the nose and ears), fibrocartilage (found in the disks between the vertebrae in the spinal cord), and hyaline cartilage (the type that protects mobile joints such as knees).

Cartilage consists of several component elements:

- Chondrocytes, the specialized cells that produce and maintain cartilage
- Collagen, the major structural protein in the body
- Proteoglycans, types of proteins that are attached to chains of sugar-based molecules known as glycosaminoglycans
- Glycoproteins, which encourage the various components to bind together
- Water

The extract mix of these components varies according to type of cartilage. In cartilage that protects joints, chondrocytes make up about 5 percent of cartilage tissue; and the remaining 95 percent of the elements form a gel-like substance that surrounds the chondrocytes. Water accounts for about 70 percent of cartilage volume. Together these components comprise a *matrix* that provides the underlying structure for cartilage.

Why Cartilage Degrades

Although cartilage is often referred to as a shock absorber, in many respects it functions more like a sponge. When you move, pressure is applied to your joints. When you walk, each step places a force equal to three times your weight on the joints involved. If you are a 130-pound woman, a leisurely walk places roughly 390 pounds of force on your ankles, knees, and hips. (Running and jumping place even more pressure on joints.) Under the force of that impact, water is squeezed out of your cartilage matrix into the space between your bones where it mixes with the synovial fluid. When your joint relaxes, your cartilage reabsorbs water. This is what gives cartilage its resiliency and helps cushion your joints against weight and pressure.

As you age, two things happen that make your joints more susceptible to injury. Your muscles tend to weaken and become tighter, providing less cushioning power to absorb pressure, and your cartilage begins to change and loses it resiliency. The once tightly woven cartilage matrix loses some of its cohesion. As a result, your cartilage begins to absorb more water. As the cartilage matrix becomes more hydrated, it loses some of its essential building blocks such as proteoglycans. The end result is a softer, less resilient structure. Your cartilage becomes more susceptible to wear and tear, which only increases the damage. A vicious cycle is set in motion that may eventually lead to the development of osteoarthritis.

Denied the protective cushion that healthy cartilage provides, your bones will feel the impact of each movement, and you may feel pain afterward. You may find your joints becoming stiff and sore gradually. If the condition worsens, your bones may actually begin to grind against each other, and small bumps known as bone spurs may develop. The pain only worsens. (See How Osteoarthritis Damages Joints.)

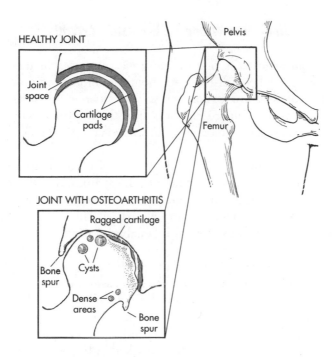

How Osteoarthritis Damages Joints

In a healthy joint like this hip joint, cartilage covers the ends of bones, reducing friction and absorbing shock. Osteoarthritis damages cartilage and allows bones to rub together. As the disease advances, bone spurs, abnormally decreased density, and cysts may develop.

Fortunately, aging in and of itself is not enough to cause osteoarthritis; otherwise, everyone would develop the disease. What will put you more at risk or protect you are your own unique characteristics. These include such things as heredity, overall health and fitness, hormonal changes, and past medical history (which includes mechanical factors such as the effects of injury or repetitive exposure to large forces). We'll discuss these factors, and what you can do to minimize your own risk, in chapter 3, Protecting Yourself.

What Goes Wrong in Rheumatoid Arthritis

Rheumatoid arthritis is one of the great mysteries in medicine. While much has been discovered about the underlying process of the disease and its progression, it is still not clear how it starts in the first place. As a result, researchers find themselves examining a number of tantalizing clues, but the true villain or villains remain unknown.

Complicating the situation is the nature of rheumatoid arthritis itself. The disease is a moving target: The symptoms and progression of the disease differ from one person to another and may even fluctuate in the same person from year to year. This makes it hard to identify disease patterns that would enable researchers to find the culprit.

This much is known: In rheumatoid arthritis the disease process begins in the synovial membrane that encases each mobile joint. This membrane produces synovial fluid, which fills the space between the bones and lubricates the joints. Only later, as rheumatoid arthritis progresses, does it affect cartilage and bone.

Ironically, rheumatoid arthritis is sparked by the very mechanism that is intended to fight illnesses and infection: the immune system.

How the Immune System Functions

The immune system is one of your best allies. Incredibly complex, it has the diversity of an ant colony, with different cells that function as sentries and soldiers, workers and managers. When your immune system works well, you'll see few visible signs of its activity—some inflammation at a cut, perhaps, or the mucus that can be so annoying during a cold. But soon the signs and symptoms disappear, and you forget all about it.

Normally your immune system provides an efficient defense system. For instance, if you cut your knee, white blood cells move quickly to the site of the injury like a fleet of ambulances. They surround any foreign material such as bacteria that has invaded through the open wound. Then, like ambulances opening their doors to release a team of emergency medical technicians, your white blood cells give rise to more specialized cells capable of performing various healing tasks. At the same time your white blood cells produce chemicals that cause your blood vessels to dilate so that more rescue cells can arrive. You will see the area turn red, and it will feel warm to the touch. It may also swell. This process is known as inflammation.

Once your wound heals or once you have successfully fought the infection, your immune system calls off its attack, and the various helpers, sentries, and soldiers dissipate. The affected area returns to normal as inflammation subsides.

How the Immune System Overreacts in Rheumatoid Arthritis

The immune system, the body's defense against foreign invaders, is indeed a *system*. It consists of a wide variety of generalists, which can be used in a number of situations, and specialists, which home in only on particular targets. One of the most striking and useful things about the immune system is that many of these players appear in great quantities when there is work to be done, and then disappear when they are no longer needed. In this respect the immune system is like a good and trusted friend: always around, on a moment's notice, when you need it.

Somehow, in rheumatoid arthritis, friends become foes. Like guests who have stayed too long at a party, having one too many drinks, they go crashing about the place, destroying things and creating a mess.

Stage 1: The Immune Response Begins. The mayhem that leads to rheumatoid arthritis begins when some still unidentified foreign agent invades the body of someone who is susceptible. The body recognizes the invader as *other*, and the immune system responds. First on the scene are sentries that are ever alert to invaders. In the synovial membrane that surrounds mobile joints, these sentries consist mainly of cells known as *macrophages*. They essentially engulf the invader, chew it into bits, and then strip off tiny fragments that can be used to identify other invaders like it. The alert is sounded.

That may appear complicated and cumbersome, but the process is actually quite elegant. One writer has called macrophages the town criers of the immune system. They sound an alert and wait for the immune system troops to arrive. Immune system sentries known as helper T cells are the first to respond. They assess the situation and decide what type of immune system soldier should be called to the scene.

Oddly enough, while all this activity is going on in the bloodstream—the macrophages engulfing the invader and sounding an alert; the helper T cells deciding which type of soldier should respond—you may not notice anything amiss. At this stage there are no symptoms.

Stage 2: The Immune Response Escalates. Now that the immune system has recognized a foreign invader, it initiates a cascade of events meant to ensure that the invader is destroyed.

The helper T cells call for the soldiers. There are two broad categories of soldiers in the immune system: *killer* T cells, which can attack an enemy head-on, and B lymphocytes, which manufacture and release antibodies specifically designed to home in on and destroy the foreign invader. Meanwhile, other changes take place to enable additional immune system cells to reach the area. The macrophages, which originally helped sound the alert about the invader, now help new blood vessels to form. They are assisted by hormonelike substances called cytokines, which enhance and amplify the process of inflammation that has now begun.

Other immune system cells that are circulating elsewhere in the body home in on the joint, attracted by all the commotion. These cells start to accumulate in the synovial membrane surrounding the joint.

Meanwhile, other immune system cells known as neutrophils, a type of white blood cell, begin to accumulate in the synovial fluid that fills the joint cavity. Neutrophils exist as a type of cleanup mechanism at the site of infection; they consume the debris of an immune system assault and any other unwanted particles or bacteria. They do this by releasing digestive substances known as lysoso-mal enzymes that break down and dissolve their targets.

At the same time another component of the immune system known as the complement system is activated. This unleashes proteins that further speed the destruction of foreign particles by antibodies.

If it is beginning to sound like a war, in some ways it is. The immune system has launched its versions of an army, a navy, and an air force in order to destroy the invader. But in rheumatoid arthritis, for reasons that remain unclear, the attack not only continues beyond the original goal of destroying the enemy but also escalates. As many as a billion neutrophils may be circulating in the synovial fluid of a knee that is moderately inflamed. The enzymes they release, once directed at a foreign invader, start to take on healthy cartilage and ligaments.

By this time you are quite aware that something is wrong. You might feel stiff upon awakening, and it may take as much as an hour to limber up. Pain will begin and intensify.

If it continues without interference, the "war" going on beneath the surface of the skin will begin to take its toll. Lost mobility, visible swelling in the joint, and, for some people, increased fatigue are the results. As the immune system assaults continue, even the bones and cartilage will be pummeled and destroyed. If the disease continues unchecked, joints may become deformed. (See Joint Changes in Rheumatoid Arthritis on page 30.)

What You Can Do to Protect Yourself

There is no way to prevent some of the damage described in this chapter. We all grow older, and our cartilage will begin to lose resiliency just as our skin begins to wrinkle. And no one knows what causes rheumatoid arthritis, which is the first step in learning how to prevent it.

But there are steps you can take to control what you can and minimize any damage that occurs. In the next several chapters we'll

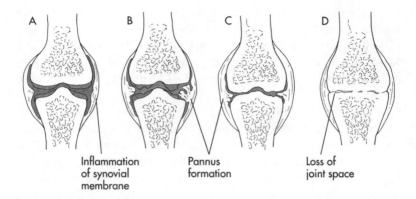

Inflammation   Pannus   Loss of
of synovial   formation   joint space
membrane

Joint Changes in Rheumatoid Arthritis

In rheumatoid arthritis, inflammation begins in the synovial membrane (A). The synovial membrane begins to proliferate and forms extra tissue called pannus *(B). Cells in the pannus release enzymes that eat into the cartilage, bone, and soft tissues (C). Finally, the tendons and joint capsule may become inflamed, causing bone damage (D).*

discuss this and how to recognize symptoms early enough to seek appropriate medical care. In all forms of arthritis, the earlier you intervene and take action, the better.

CHAPTER 3

Protecting Yourself

"So now they tell me," Sue thought as she read the article about arthritis. Ten or fifteen years ago it was "no pain, no gain" and "feel the burn." And she had taken that advice to heart when she started running in her thirties. She really pushed herself, really pounded the pavement. And if her joints ached occasionally, that was the way it was supposed to be, right?

But this article claimed that exercises such as running could damage her knee joints. And regular typing at a computer keyboard was another no-no.

Could it be that all the pounding her joints had taken over the years might have hurt her in some way? Sue had reason to wonder. Now forty-two, she was beginning to feel stiff when she got up the morning after a long run. Sometimes at work her back ached while working at her computer. In trying to become physically fit, had she inadvertently put herself at risk of arthritis? And if so, what could she do to reverse the damage and prevent additional injury?

WE CHANGE as we get older. We like to think we become wiser. We hate to think about wrinkles. And unless we do something about it, we become weaker and more susceptible to all sorts of injury, including arthritis.

Bones may thin in a process known as osteoporosis—where the bone literally becomes more porous. Muscles weaken, and tendons can shorten and tighten. All this has an impact on the health of our joints.

One study by researchers at the Indiana University School of Medicine showed that overweight women with weak thigh muscles were more likely than other women to develop osteoarthritis later in life. The study concluded that the women's obesity was putting undue strain on their joints, and their muscles were not able to provide proper support and stability to counteract this stress.

The best way to reduce the risk of developing arthritis, or at least minimize the debilitating effects, is to learn more about how to maintain your health and protect your joints. Better attention to diet, fitness, and exercise, especially as you grow older, is a good way to start. More information about good nutrition, specific exercises, and protective shoes and other equipment are included in the following pages.

And if you have already developed arthritis, there are still steps you can take to ensure that your condition does not worsen. Check with your healthcare provider to develop an individual strategy. Some of the exercise and diet tips provided in this chapter may be of use if your arthritis is mild. For moderate and more severe forms of arthritis, read about diet and exercise in chapter 12.

What Puts You at Risk for Arthritis

Arthritis is similar to other serious diseases, such as heart disease and cancer, which develop because of a complex interplay of heredity, biology, and environmental factors.

Heredity

If members of your immediate family (grandparents, parents, or siblings) have arthritis, then you are more likely to develop the disease than if none of your immediate relatives are affected. The susceptibility to both osteoarthritis and rheumatoid arthritis seems to run in families. This is a risk factor you cannot change, but you should be aware of it so that you can take steps to protect yourself.

Biology

Biology is a broad term that encompasses a range of factors, including age, gender, hormones, weight, activities, and genetic profile. Some factors can be changed; others cannot. Acting together, all these characteristics might make you more or less susceptible to certain diseases, including arthritis.

Take your genetic profile, for example. It is easy to think of genes as static and unchanging; this perception may be reinforced by news accounts that begin, "A gene has been found . . ." Such reports make it seem as if genes are heavy and solid, like paperweights; in fact, they are much more interesting and dynamic.

Each of us has twenty-six chromosomes and roughly fifty thousand genes. (More about these genes will be known when the Human Genome Project, which seeks to identify every gene in our bodies, has progressed further.) These genes are like how-to books in a library: They provide detailed instructions on how to make enzymes and proteins, the building blocks of the body. Genes provide instructions about our hair color, how tall we will grow, and how fair or dark our skin will be. But they also govern many less visible aspects of our bodies, including the function of our immune system and our susceptibility to developing certain diseases. Some scientists think that if you develop osteoarthritis, you may have a gene or set of genes that makes your cartilage more prone to damage. If you do not develop osteoarthritis, you may have a protective form of the gene.

Environment

"Environment" is another scientific term that can be confusing and is sometimes misinterpreted. After all, the word conjures up images of the great outdoors.

When used by healthcare providers, "environment" refers to anything outside the body such as diet, previous injury to a joint, exposure to infection, choice of profession, and choice of leisure activities. All these may contribute to the development of arthritis, especially if you already have an inherited or biologic susceptibility to the disease.

Working in an office can be particularly hazardous to muscles and joints, for instance. We slouch in our chairs, spend hours sitting in the same position, pound away at our keyboards, and twist our spines into unreasonable positions as we cradle a phone against our ears and take notes. This can cause muscles to tighten and shorten and joints to become stiff.

Some environmental factors can be changed.

Risk Factors for Osteoarthritis

A number of risk factors increase your chances of developing osteoarthritis, especially if you are already susceptible for some other reason such as family history of the disease. You can take steps to reduce your chances of developing osteoarthritis by avoiding the risks you can control.

Age. Your risk of developing osteoarthritis increases with age. Most people who develop the disease are middle-aged or older, and the incidence increases exponentially after the age of fifty. It is not clear why age is such a big risk factor. As discussed in chapter 2, cartilage in the joints begins to wear out as we age. But your joints are also remarkably resilient, and the challenge as you grow older is to find ways to provide extra protection for your joints as they become more vulnerable.

Obesity. If you are overweight, you are increasing your risk of developing osteoarthritis because of the extra strain placed on your joints, especially the weight-bearing joints such as the knees. Obesity can also worsen osteoarthritis once it has developed. Shedding excess pounds may reduce your chances of developing osteoarthritis. If you already have the disease, losing weight will help prevent it from becoming worse.

Genetic profile. As with many diseases, you are more likely to develop osteoarthritis if you have an immediate family member—grandparent, parent, or sibling—who has developed the disease. Researchers have identified at least one gene involved in a distinct subtype of osteoarthritis, and it is likely they will soon develop others involved in other forms of the disease. But having such an inherited predisposition does not guarantee that you will develop the disease, just that you are more prone to developing it. If you have a family history of osteoarthritis, you may want to pay special attention to controlling other risk factors to reduce your chances of developing the disease.

Injury. If your joint becomes injured or infected, that may increase your chances of developing osteoarthritis in the joint later on. The initial insult may damage the cartilage and other joint tissues in some way, setting in motion the deterioration that ultimately results in osteoarthritis. Many cases of osteoarthritis in the knee, for instance, develop in the years following a knee injury.

Hormones. Levels of hormones, particularly estrogen, may affect the development of osteoarthritis. Researchers have found that in older age groups the prevalence of osteoarthritis is higher in women than in men. Moreover, it may affect multiple joints and be more severe. If you are a woman approaching menopause or have already gone through it, ask your healthcare provider about the risks and benefits of hormone replacement therapy. Some studies have suggested that this therapy helps protect against the development of some types of osteoarthritis. The exact reasons remain unclear but may have something to do with the way estrogen regulates the normal maintenance of bones and cartilage.

Too much activity. Experts are divided about whether too much physical activity and exercise, whether on the job or recreationally, increase your chances of developing osteoarthritis.

Some researchers have found that if you overuse a joint, especially in a physically demanding way, you will be more likely to develop osteoarthritis in that joint later on; for instance, construction workers who operate heavy machinery such as jack hammers, may be more at risk for developing osteoarthritis in their hands. And some studies have reported greater incidence of osteoarthritis in former elite athletes than in the general population.

But other investigators are not so sure. They have found that most people who work or exercise are no more likely to develop osteoarthritis because of the pressure that activity puts on their joints. For instance, one nine-year study of longtime runners found they were no more likely than nonrunners to develop osteoarthritis. Another study that involved a group of men who ran an average of twenty-eight miles per week for twelve years also found no greater incidence of diagnosed osteoarthritis than in nonrunners.

Given such evidence, some researchers conclude that our joints are remarkably resilient even when exposed to repeated low-impact exercise or motions. Osteoarthritis will develop only when normal joints are repeatedly exposed to high-level impact or have become susceptible because of previous injury, misalignment, or other types of biological vulnerability.

Inactivity. Ironically, too little activity may also put you at risk. If you exercise only once in a while, you can lose flexibility in your joints. The muscles around the joints may weaken, increasing the chances of injury. Once you develop osteoarthritis, inactivity can worsen symptoms, especially stiffness. That is why physical therapy is such an important part of your treatment plan (see chapter 10).

Certainly maintaining physical fitness while taking common-sense steps to protect your joints can only improve your overall health.

Risk Factors for Rheumatoid Arthritis

As discussed in chapter 2, rheumatoid arthritis is a medical mystery. Even so, researchers have identified several factors that appear to increase risk.

Genetic profile. It is likely that we inherit genes that make us more or less susceptible to rheumatoid arthritis. The suspect genes are those that regulate the immune system. A prevailing theory of the cause of rheumatoid arthritis is that it develops only after some environmental factor—an injury, hormones, or an infection—is added to the underlying susceptibility.

This theory has gained support since a genetic marker, HLA-DR4, was found in the blood of many people who have rheumatoid arthritis. Although the gene or genes involved have not yet been identified, many researchers expect it is only a matter of time.

Gender factors. Because rheumatoid arthritis is two to three times more common in women than in men, many researchers suspect that some aspect of gender difference plays a role in the development of this disease. This theory is borne out by preliminary findings of several studies. Although none of these observations are conclusive, they provide interesting clues.

- Women who are fifty or younger—that is, premenopausal—are much more likely than men to develop rheumatoid arthritis. After age fifty the differences are not as pronounced.
- Three out of four women with rheumatoid arthritis who get pregnant have their disease go into remission until they give birth.

Much more research needs to be done in this area to clarify the impact of gender on the development of rheumatoid arthritis.

Infection. One popular theory holds that an infectious agent somehow triggers a misguided immune response in susceptible people who then develop rheumatoid arthritis. This theory has gained further support since the infectious agent responsible for Lyme disease, which can cause a form of arthritis similar to rheumatoid arthritis, has been identified. (For more information about Lyme disease, see chapter 8.)

If there is an infectious agent involved in rheumatoid arthritis, it remains unknown, but over the years several candidates, including a variety of viruses, have been suspected. The Epstein-Barr virus, which causes infectious mononucleosis, is one leading suspect in rheumatoid arthritis. Most people with rheumatoid arthritis have antibodies in their blood that are directed against the Epstein-Barr virus (although it is also true that many people without rheumatoid arthritis have these antibodies). The virus is known to activate B lymphocytes, which in turn overproduce substances, including the one known as the rheumatoid factor that is detected in the blood of eight out of ten people with the disease. The Epstein-Barr virus is also found more often in people with rheumatoid arthritis than in those who do not have the disease. We do not know, however, if the Epstein-Barr virus is involved actively in rheumatoid arthritis, nor have we yet identified any specific infections as a cause for this disease.

What You Can Do to Protect Your Joints

You can't control everything in your life, and certainly you can't change some of the factors that put you at risk for developing arthritis. But it is possible to take steps to protect your joints and maintain your overall well-being—and thereby prevent avoidable damage and lessen the impact of the disease should it occur.

To maintain health the prescription is deceptively easy: Eat right and exercise regularly. You've heard this advice before, but it bears repeating—especially when it comes to arthritis.

A healthy diet is one that provides the nutrients you need for your body to function efficiently. Too much of the wrong foods provide "garbage" calories that add weight without contributing to function. And as mentioned earlier in this chapter, excess weight places undue pressure on joints and can increase your risk for certain types of arthritis.

Exercise is important as well. As we get older, our muscles weaken and tendons shrink. This makes us more prone to injury. It also means we are less able to provide the type of support our joints need to withstand the routine pounding they take every day. Fortunately, when it comes to exercise, we can "turn back the clock." With the right fitness plan you can rejuvenate your muscles and restore the strength and tone you may have lost.

In the pages that follow we'll explore diet and exercise as a way of protecting your overall health and your joints as much as possible.

The Myth of the Arthritis Diet

We're sure you've heard about an arthritis diet from some well-intentioned friend or perhaps in the pages of a magazine or book. So before we go into detail about what comprises a healthy diet, we want to put the myth of an arthritis diet to rest.

As discussed in chapter 2, arthritis consists of more than one hundred different conditions. So far, only one of them—gout—has been linked to what you eat. People with gout have too much uric acid in their bloodstream. This acid results when you digest meats or fish that contain purines. In gout, people either make too much uric acid or are unable to flush it out through the kidneys and urine. As a result, the uric acid crystallizes and accumulates in joints, causing pain and inflammation (see chapter 8 for more information on gout).

Healthcare providers sometimes recommend that people with gout avoid foods that contain purines: meat, poultry, dried beans and peas, fish such as anchovies, herring, scallops, and certain vegetables. They may also advise them to flush the uric acid out of their system by drinking a lot of water and to avoid alcohol, which raises uric acid levels in the blood.

But the dietary link to other forms of arthritis is not as clear. Certainly some people are allergic to some foods, and this might worsen the pain and symptoms of arthritis. And there are some foods, such as the omega-3 fatty acids found in cold-water fish like mackerel and salmon, that enable you to fight inflammation, which can be a factor in certain types of arthritis.

Still, the evidence so far is scarce that any diet change in and of itself will help protect you against arthritis. As the research continues, we think the best advice is to eat a healthy, well-balanced diet. That will improve your overall well-being and assist you in staying healthy for as long as possible.

The Components of a Healthy Diet

As you digest food, it is broken down into nutrients that are absorbed into your bloodstream and carried to every cell in your body. Your body needs about forty different nutrients every day to keep you healthy.

Water. Often overlooked as a nutrient, water is actually essential to your health. It transports nutrients throughout your body and flushes away waste products. To maintain good health you should drink eight large glasses of liquids—ideally, water—every day. That may seem like a lot, but other liquids—alcohol, coffee, and some types of soda—are diuretics that rid your body of water, so it's important to keep yourself hydrated.

Carbohydrates. These are found in such foods as bread, pasta, rice, dried beans and peas, potatoes, cereals, sugars, fruits, and vegetables. Recent studies indicate that obtaining carbohydrates through eating whole-grain foods (as opposed to "refined" grains) is better for sustained good health and offers protection against a variety of chronic diseases.

Fiber. Found only in plant foods, fiber provides the bulk necessary to help your large intestine move waste out of your system. A diet high in fiber prevents constipation and may be associated with a lower risk of heart disease, type 2 diabetes, and diverticular disease. Experts recommend that you consume at least 25 grams of fiber every day. Check the nutrition labels to find out how much fiber a particular food contains. A bowl of fortified bran cereal (two cups), for instance, contains 10 grams of fiber. A cup of frozen chopped kale contains 6 grams. A half-cup of brown rice contains 2 grams. Fresh fruits and vegetables also contain varying amounts of fiber. Try to eat a variety of plant foods throughout the day, and you'll consume enough fiber.

Fats and oils. Some dietary fats are better for your health than others. Try to avoid fats and oils that contain high levels of cholesterol, saturated fats, and trans-saturated fats, such as those found in fatty meats, whole milk, vegetable shortenings, margarine, and many commercially baked goods. Instead, consume foods with polyunsaturated or monounsaturated fats, such as those found in natural vegetable oils.

Some foods, such as fish and flaxseed oil, contain substances known as omega-3 fatty acids. Although more research needs to be done, the omega-3 fatty acids appear to be of value in the treatment of some forms of heart disease and arthritis.

Proteins. Proteins help build, repair, and maintain body tissue. This nutrient is found in meat, poultry, fish, eggs, milk, cheese, yogurt, and soy products, as well as beans, seeds, nuts, and, in smaller amounts, grain products and many vegetables. Although protein is helpful, try not to overdo it. Too much protein, particularly animal protein, may actually contribute to such conditions as bone loss. About 10 to 15 percent of your daily caloric intake should be protein. Anything above that will only be flushed out in your urine.

Vitamins and minerals. Your body cannot make vitamins, so it is important that you consume some every day. There are thirteen essential vitamins, and each has a specific role in keeping you healthy. There is strong evidence that people who eat a lot of vitamin-rich foods, such as vegetables, fruits, and whole grains, are in better health than those who do not.

Minerals help regulate fluid balance, muscle contractions, and nerve impulses, and are essential for the development of bones and teeth. There are at least twenty minerals in a balanced diet, including calcium, magnesium, sodium, iron, potassium, and phosphorous. Major minerals such as calcium are needed to build bones in childhood and slow the rate of bone loss in adulthood to prevent the bone-thinning condition of osteoporosis. Like vitamins, the best way to get the minerals needed for health is by eating a balanced diet rich in fruits, vegetables, and whole grains.

Women, who are especially vulnerable to osteoporosis, should have 1,000 to 1,500 milligrams of calcium every day, depending on age and any medications they may be taking. Teenage girls should consume this much calcium in order to build up as much bone mass as possible. Additionally, recent evidence suggests that increasing vitamin D along with calcium may be an effective way to prevent bone loss. If you don't get enough calcium and vitamin D from your diet, try supplements.

For more information about the components of a healthy diet, see our companion book, *The Harvard Medical School Family Health Guide.*

What to Eat Every Day

The U.S. Department of Health and Human Services and the Department of Agriculture have developed dietary guidelines that

offer specific recommendations on what people should eat to maximize their health and help reduce the risk of certain chronic diseases. In general, you should

- Maintain a healthy weight to reduce your risk of having
  high blood pressure, heart disease, a stroke, certain types of
  cancer (including postmenopausal breast cancer and
  cancers of the uterus, colon, and kidney) and also to reduce
  your risk of type 2 diabetes, infertility, arthritis, gallstones,
  snoring, or sleep apnea.
- Eat a variety of foods to get the energy, protein, vitamins,
  minerals, and fiber needed for good health.
- Choose a diet low in saturated fat, trans-saturated fat, and
  cholesterol—or substitute monounsaturated or
  polyunsaturated fats whenever possible—to reduce your
  risk of obesity and heart disease.
- Choose a diet with plenty of fruits, vegetables, and whole
  grain products, which provide needed vitamins, minerals,
  fiber, and complex carbohydrates.
- Use sugars only in moderation to curb weight gain and
  prevent dental cavities.
- Use salt only in moderation to help prevent high blood
  pressure, a risk factor for heart disease.
- Drink alcoholic beverages only in moderation because
  alcohol supplies calories but few or no nutrients. One drink
  per day may have a protective effect against heart disease.
  Do not drink any alcohol if you are pregnant.
- Eat a maximum of 4 ounces of lean meat, skinless poultry,
  or fish once or twice a day; this provides all needed protein.

The Importance of Exercise

Diet alone cannot keep you healthy. Regular exercise is also
required to promote overall well-being and build strong muscles,
and to ensure that you are providing as much support to your joints
as possible.

A regular fitness plan will help to

- Strengthen your heart, enabling it to pump blood more efficiently throughout your body (carrying much needed nutrients and oxygen)
- Improve levels of cholesterol in your blood by lowering harmful LDL cholesterol and increasing "good" HDL cholesterol
- Increase your breathing capacity
- strengthen your bones by slowing the process of bone thinning known as osteoporosis
- Strengthen your muscles and provide more support to your joints
- Decrease your blood pressure
- Reduce your risk of developing chronic illnesses such as diabetes and heart disease
- Possibly protect against some types of cancer

In many instances a regular exercise plan will help you lose weight, which in turn takes the pressure off your joints. To shed pounds you need to expend more calories than you consume each day. The best way to lose weight is to begin slowly, aiming for no more than 2 pounds per week. And what you do eat should be healthy food, such as fruits, vegetables, and whole grains.

But regular exercise will help you do more than just lose weight. It increases your endurance and helps you digest foods more readily and sleep better at night. It also enables you to withstand stress and anxiety, and will make you less likely to become depressed. All these factors will enable you to cope better with the symptoms of arthritis should they occur.

Regular exercise also benefits your joints directly. As discussed in chapter 2, your muscles and tendons help align your bones and absorb the sometimes impressive amounts of force placed on your joints every day. If you lose weight and build muscle, you will provide further support to your joints.

Physical Fitness

To become physically fit, start slowly—perhaps only ten or fifteen minutes a day. Then try to build up gradually over a few months so that you are exercising at least thirty minutes a day. Take your time; this will help you from becoming discouraged, enabling you to build muscle and aerobic capacity safely so that you don't hurt yourself. Even moderate activity can benefit your muscles, as seen in Major Muscle Groups and Everyday Activities in Which They Are Used.

A good fitness plan consists of aerobic, strength, and flexibility exercises. These will be explored in the pages that follow.

Warming Up and Cooling Down

Whether you are in shape or trying to become more physically fit, experts advise that you warm up before exercising and cool down afterward. This prepares your body for exercise in a gradual fashion and decreases the chances of unintended injury such as a pulled muscle. Warm-up exercises also literally raise the temperature in your muscles and joints so that they function more efficiently and are less prone to injury while exercising.

The best way to warm up is to start your intended activity slowly. Continue the activity for about five minutes, until your body begins to feel warm and more limber. Then you can do a series of stretching exercises, focusing on those muscles that you intend to exercise (that is, if you are going to run, stretch your leg muscles especially). See the section below on flexibility exercises for some suggestions.

After you have completed your exercise routine, it is likely that you will feel warm (maybe even sweaty) and your heart will be beating fast. Then it's time to cool down—literally. You can cool down by repeating the gentle stretching exercises you used earlier to warm up. A cool-down period enables your breathing and body temperature to return to normal gradually and also reduces your risk of having sore muscles the next day.

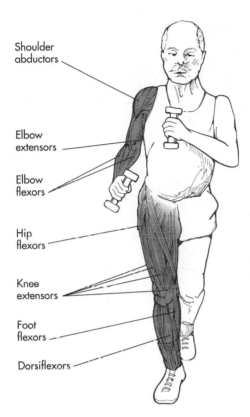

Shoulder
abductors

Elbow
extensors

Elbow
flexors

Hip
flexors

Knee
extensors

Foot
flexors

Dorsiflexors

Stair Climbing
Knee extensors
Hip extensors and flexors
Foot flexors
Dorsiflexors
Knee flexors and extensors
Hip flexors

Walking
Knee extensors
Hip extensors and flexors
Knee flexors and extensors
Dorsiflexors
Foot flexors

Getting Up from a Chair
Shoulder abductors
Elbow extensors
Knee extensors
Hip extensors and flexors
Dorsiflexors

Reaching
Shoulder abductors
Elbow extensors

Lifting, Carrying
Elbow flexors
Shoulder abductors

Major Muscle Groups and Everyday Activities in Which They Are Used

You may not realize it, but you use all your major muscle groups during the course of a normal day. Even moderate activity, such as brisk walking, carrying your groceries, or taking the stairs, has a beneficial impact on muscle groups

Flexibility Exercises

Exercises that improve flexibility help keep you limber and improve your range of motion. When you extend your arm or turn your head to look at something, notice how easily and how far you are able to move the joints involved. If you feel stiff and aren't able to move as easily as you once did, don't worry. Your muscles have tightened, perhaps because you've been in a sedentary job or because you have been trying to exercise but have not focused on flexibility. Fortunately, it is possible to increase flexibility by stretching the muscles that surround the joint. In fact, studies have shown that no matter how old you are, you can improve your flexibility.

Flexibility exercises stretch muscle groups. As the muscles extend, your body becomes more limber and you are better able to take the impact of exercise. Flexibility exercises are helpful when warming up or cooling down.

The easiest way to build flexibility is to do gentle and slow stretches every day. In general it's best to do the following:

- Stretch as far as you can and then hold the position for a few seconds. Don't bob up and down; that can pull a muscle. It's better to stretch in a slow, fluid motion.
- Stretch a little bit further but not so much that it hurts. Hold the second position for twenty to thirty seconds. (If you do not hold the position for at least twenty seconds, it won't do you any good; it takes that long to increase flexibility.)
- Relax and return to your starting position.
- If you have a hard time keeping your balance while stretching, either hold on to something for support or gaze at a fixed object in the distance; this will help your body maintain its own balance.
- Try to stay relaxed as you stretch. Continue to breathe and even try to breathe a little deeper, which will relax you.

To get started on your flexibility exercise plan, try the exercises illustrated in the following Flexibility Exercises.

Flexibility Exercises

For Triceps

Sit or stand upright with your left arm behind your lower back, placed as far up your back as possible. Hold a rolled-up towel in your right hand, lift your right arm overhead, and bend your right elbow so that your right arm hangs down your back. Grasp the towel with your left hand. Work your hands together. Hold the stretch for 10 seconds, then relax. Reverse arm positions and repeat.

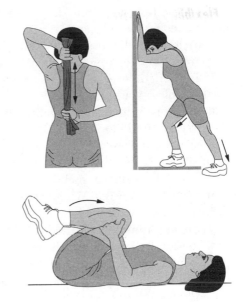

For Calf and Achilles Tendon

Stand upright, slightly more than an arm's length from a wall. Place your right leg forward, keeping the left leg straight. Lean against the wall with your lower arms flat against the wall. Keep the heel of your left (back) foot down with the sole flat on the floor and the toes pointing forward. Hold the stretch for 10 seconds, then relax. Switch legs and repeat.

For Lower Back

Lie flat on your back. Bend both knees and slide your feet toward your buttocks. Grasp your thighs and pull your knees toward your chest, elevating your hips slightly. Hold the stretch for 30 seconds. Straighten your legs slowly, one at a time.

Flexibility exercises help you warm up and cool down after a workout. Stretch gently, never pushing yourself to the point where you feel pain.

Resistance Exercises

Resistance exercises strengthen muscles, which in turn provide better support and protection to joints. It's actually possible to become stronger than you were when you were younger. One study showed that women and men aged seventy-two to ninety-eight could triple their leg strength by doing resistance exercises. They also walked faster and gained range of motion in their knees.

Muscle strength is easy to take for granted. As we grow older, we also grow stronger—until the age of about thirty to forty, when muscle strength levels off. At that point your muscles will become weaker unless you do something to keep them strong. It is likely that you won't notice you're getting weaker, but you might notice that you get tired more easily, find activities like mowing the lawn harder to do, and are more likely to pull a muscle.

In strength training you strengthen muscles by working against some type of resistance, such as that provided by lifting weights or lifting your leg in water. When you do such exercises for twenty to thirty minutes, two or three times a week, you actually build muscle.

There are simple ways to add weight training to your daily activities. You can strap ankle or wrist weights when you walk, or you can carry hand weights. You can even do something as simple as lifting canned goods while in the kitchen. If you have access to a pool, you can exercise in the water, using the water to provide resistance that will not hurt your joints.

The key in strength training is in repeating the motion (sometimes called doing "reps" in fitness clubs). When exercising a particular muscle, repeat the motion for eight to twelve times before increasing the weight or resistance you are working against. (If you cannot yet do eight repetitions, decrease the weight or resistance.)

Some simple ways to add resistance to your exercise plan:

- Use your own body weight to create resistance by doing such things as push-ups or sit-ups (but protect your back while doing sit-ups by bending your legs at the knees).
- Use free weights such as hand and ankle weights or even canned goods from the kitchen.
- Working on exercise machines creates resistance, but if you don't have access to a health club, you can also try using latex stretch bands. Available in many sports stores, these extend and retract as you apply and release pressure while you do exercises.

When you do strengthening exercises, try not to "lock" your joints. Rather, extend the joint involved almost but not quite as far as it can go. For instance, leave your elbow or knee bent slightly before returning to the starting position. This avoids injury.

Move slowly and fluidly, much as you do when stretching. And when you're finished with your strength training routine, take a day off. Muscles need from two to three days of rest before being exercised again to ensure that they become stronger.

See below for some examples of resistance exercises you can try on your own.

Aerobic Exercises

Resistance Exercises

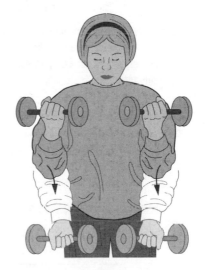

Hold a 1-pound hand weight (or soup can) in each hand. Stand with your back straight, knees slightly apart. With your palms facing upward, hold the weights at thigh level. Lift the weights slowly up toward your chest. Lower them again to thigh level. Do this with controlled, slow movements. When you can repeat this exercise 12 times, increase your weights by 1-pound increments.
Strength exercises require moving small groups of muscles only a few times against a degree of resistance. Strength training, which is done to improve muscle mass, may be dynamic—such as weight lifting, in which the muscles actually change in length—or isometric, in which the muscles contract without shortening and are briefly tensed using one part of the body to resist the movement of another part.

Aerobic exercises increase your endurance and energy levels by increasing your heart and breathing rates so that more oxygen and nutrients are circulated through the body. This type of exercise also benefits your bones and muscles.

Whenever you exercise so that your heart rate rises above its resting level, your heart and lungs benefit. To achieve maximum benefit, try to do some type of aerobic exercise for at least thirty minutes a day, five days a week, working hard enough to reach your target rate. A handy rule of thumb is to exercise vigorously enough so that, after about ten minutes, you can talk but not sing while exercising.

Target Heart Rate Zone

To measure your heart rate after exercising vigorously, locate your pulse in your wrist or neck and count the number of beats you feel during a 10-second interval. Multiply that number by 6 to calculate your heart rate per minute. To determine your target heart rate zone:

1. Subtract your age from the number 220. The answer is your predicted maximum heart rate.
2. Multiply your predicted maximum heart rate (the answer to Step 1) by .55. This number represents the low end of your heart rate range.
3. Multiply your predicted maximum heart rate (the answer to Step 1) by .85. This number represents the high end of your heart rate range.

For example, if you are 40 years old, then your predicted maximum heart rate is $220 - 40 = 180$. Therefore, the low end of the range for you is $180 \times .55$ (or 99 beats per minute), and the high end is $180 \times .85$ (or 153 beats per minute).

Some examples of aerobic activities include:

- Swimming
- Walking fast
- Running
- Bicycling
- Climbing stairs
- Skipping rope

- Playing tennis
- Hiking
- Mowing the lawn with a push mower

Building an Exercise Program

Although you should start your exercise program slowly, most experts advise aiming for a goal of thirty minutes of moderate physical activity per day on most days of the week. A brisk walk or mowing the lawn are two examples of moderate physical activity. But remember there are three aspects to physical fitness, and a good exercise plan will include a mix of each one every week:

FLEXIBILITY EXERCISES	3 to 5 minutes per day, best done before exercising, and 5 to 10 minutes after exercising
AEROBIC EXERCISES	30 minutes most days (can be done in increments of at least 10 minutes)
RESISTANCE EXERCISES	15 to 20 minutes at least twice a week

These recommendations are general, of course, and as you improve your physical conditioning, you may want to move beyond the minimum required.

Commonsense Strategies to Protect Your Joints

Beyond eating right and exercising regularly, we also advise a little common sense to protect your joints. As mentioned in chapter 2, every time we take a step we place approximately three times our weight on the joints in our lower extremities. The older we get, the less resilient our joints become. And while you may have been able to run a 10-mile road race in battered sneakers in your twenties, we don't advise doing the same in your forties and later. Even if you are in terrific shape, your knees need more support than those battered sneakers can provide.

Wear sensible shoes. Does this sound like advice your mother might give you? Well, Mom was right. Shoes that provide adequate support, that enable you to walk without your ankles wobbling, are the type to buy. Look for low, wide heels and designs that provide ample room for your toes.

Try to avoid high heels (higher than 2 inches) no matter how wide they are. High heels shift your body's weight away from your ankles and onto your hips and the inner part of your knee joint, which is more susceptible to wear and tear. This type of shoe also helps cause back problems and may shorten your calf muscles, making you more prone to injuries. Some orthopedists speculate that the reason women are twice as likely to develop osteoarthritis of the knee is that they wear high heels.

When it comes to sports and recreation, look for shoes that provide even more support to help you withstand the pounding on your joints. Fortunately, many stores now offer sneakers designed for walking or running. Typically, these have added support in the ankle and arch areas. (To find out more about how to protect your feet, contact organizations listed in appendix A.)

If you have a sedentary job, get up and move. As mentioned earlier in this chapter, office work can worsen the natural effects of aging. If we sit in the same place all day, our muscles become weaker, our tendons tighten, and our joints get even less support. What's the solution? Get up and move. Walk away from the desk at least once an hour. Or take ten or fifteen minutes every day to do some simple stretching exercises. Either get your coworkers to join you or close the door and tell them you're in a meeting while you do the exercises on your own.

Switch to low-impact exercises. To protect your joints and yet remain physically fit, you may want to change the type of exercise you do. Running, high-impact aerobics, and even tennis and racquetball may put a lot of strain on your joints. If you are starting to feel sore after exercising, consider switching to low-impact exercises such as bicycling and swimming. Some local health clubs even offer water aerobics classes in which you work against the resistance provided by water in the pool. This has aerobic benefits without hurting your joints.

If you are a dedicated runner and just can't give it up, make sure your shoes provide adequate support. Try to avoid running on pavement and instead run on grass or even sand (if you're lucky enough to live near a beach). These softer surfaces will cushion each step you take and lessen the impact on your joints.

Listen to your body. A number of healthcare providers have noticed a new condition dubbed "boomeritis." No, it's not a form of arthritis; it is an indication that people can get so enthused about exercise that they wind up hurting themselves. Boomeritis refers to the increasing number of muscle, tendon, and ligament injuries that healthcare providers are seeing in aging baby boomers. The way to prevent such injuries is to recognize that as you get older, you have to spend more time stretching your muscles and tendons, which have tightened with age. It's also wise to start slow, as described earlier in this chapter.

Perhaps most important, listen to your body. If you are sore for more than an hour or so after a workout has ended, you may have overdone it. Or it may be time to switch exercises to something that puts less stress on your joints. As we grow older, we have to behave more like turtles and less like hares. Just remember that in the old children's story, it was the turtle who won the race in the end.

CHAPTER 4

Getting Help

This didn't feel like the type of pain John sometimes felt when he overdid his workout at the gym. It was deep-seated, a dull ache that went away only after he sat down for a few hours. Could it be arthritis?

Helen felt stiff in the morning and not as well rested as she used to feel after a good night's sleep. She sometimes stumbled when she got out of bed. Could this be arthritis?

Once energetic and athletic, Mary was now all worn out by noon. She barely had the energy to make it through the work day, never mind go to her health club afterward. And lately she felt stiff in the morning, and one of her knees was swollen. What was this?

IF THE theme of the last chapter was "take care of yourself," then the theme of this chapter is "learn how to seek help."

Taking charge of your treatment is important. If you are diagnosed with arthritis, you will likely find yourself deluged with options and opinions—and not just from your healthcare provider. Medical information has proliferated in newspapers, magazines, bookstores, and on the Internet. Not all of the information is reliable. In this chapter we hope to provide you with the knowledge and tools to evaluate new treatments on your own. It's not that we expect you to become a healthcare professional yourself after reading this chapter, but we do want to empower you to ask intelligent questions.

Recognizing the Early Warning Signs

No matter how much you educate yourself about your joints, no matter how well you try to protect yourself against arthritis, you may still develop the disease. If so, the earlier you seek help, the better. As with many other medical conditions, treatment is much more effective if it begins soon after the disease is discovered.

As mentioned in chapter 2, typical symptoms of arthritis include fatigue, pain, stiff joints, and swelling around the joints. Ah, but how do you differentiate a normal ache or pain from one that could signal the start of arthritis? Because many forms of arthritis are slow to develop, the early symptoms are subtle. But, in general, the following guidelines will help you become more alert to the early warning signs.

Duration of symptoms. If you notice you are feeling such things as pain, stiffness, and fatigue for a longer period than you used to, this could be an early sign. Perhaps you always felt a little stiff when you got up from your desk at work to go to lunch, but if you still feel stiff by the time you reach the corner deli, a good ten-minute walk, it may be more than just desk cramps.

Intensity of symptoms. There are degrees of soreness, pain, and stiffness. As we age, we tend to get stiffer after sitting in one place for a long time. But you may notice that the mild stiffness you felt when getting out of a chair has turned into a more pronounced stiffness that makes it difficult to get out of the chair. Or maybe you not only feel stiff when getting out of bed, but actually stumble.

The same is true of fatigue. Perhaps you've always felt you had little energy in the middle of the afternoon, the so-called 3 o'clock slump. Usually you got a second wind on the way home (don't we all?). But lately you've felt worn out by lunchtime and wondered if you could make it through the day without a nap.

When sensations you have always felt suddenly become more pronounced, this may be a sign of arthritis.

New symptoms. If you notice some new symptoms, it is best to pay attention. Perhaps your right knee has begun to swell (a swollen joint that is warm to the touch is a common symptom in certain kinds of arthritis). Or perhaps you suddenly lose weight without trying. You suffer sudden bouts of fevers and chills without knowing why. Any of these could be signs of early arthritis or a number of other disorders that should be evaluated by a healthcare professional.

Where to Turn for Help

Should you suspect arthritis, the best thing to do is make an appointment with your healthcare professional.

In many cases your primary healthcare provider (a primary care physician, nurse practitioner, or physician's assistant) can diagnose arthritis. But if such a diagnosis is not made and the symptoms continue, consider visiting a rheumatologist. These specialists have advanced training in diseases affecting the joints, bones, and connective tissues. Depending on the severity of your disease, other health professionals, such as nurse specialists and physical and occupational therapists, may also assist in your care.

Health Professionals Involved in Arthritis Management

Doctors

Primary care doctors. Primary care doctors include internists and family physicians. They do not specialize in a particular field but rather are trained to recognize a broad array of illnesses and conditions. With the advent of managed care, primary care doctors are often the ones who are known as gatekeepers: They refer the patient to specialists as needed.

Internists. These doctors specialize in the diagnosis and treatment of a wide range of conditions and diseases in adults. As primary care doctors, internists can provide referrals to specialists.

Rheumatologists. These specialists are internists who have had advanced training in the care of people with diseases affecting the joints, muscles, and connective tissues such as skin and blood vessels. You may be referred to a rheumatologist by a primary care physician or internist for further evaluation and treatment.

Orthopedic surgeons. Orthopedics is a surgical specialty concerned with the bones and joints as well as the muscles, tendons, and ligaments attached to them. Orthopedic surgeons are able to perform specialized surgery to repair joints if necessary.

Rehabilitation physiatrists. Physiatrists are trained to oversee physical therapy and rehabilitation, and often work closely with other doctors and nurses.

Other Healthcare Professionals

Chiropractors. These practitioners manipulate the spinal column in therapy, based on their belief that misaligned vertebrae are the cause of many forms of illness. Although mainstream medicine disputes this underlying philosophy of disease, chiropractors can help reduce the pain associated with arthritis in the spine.

Nurse specialists or nurse practitioners. These nurses have received advanced training in various fields, including arthritis and orthopedics. They help to educate you about the condition and help with your treatment program.

Occupational therapists. These professionals work with you to find ways to reduce the wear and tear on your joints during daily activities at work or home. Special attention is paid to joints in the hands and arms.

Pharmacists. Most often seen as the people who fill prescriptions, pharmacists are capable of much more. They can explain how medications work and what the side effects might include—and, if possible, how to lessen them.

Physical therapists. These health professionals work with you to retain as much mobility as possible, even with arthritis. They may focus on exercises to strengthen muscles or advise you about how to eat better. Like nurses and occupational therapists, they may also take a lead role in educating you about arthritis and giving you self-management tips.

What Will Happen During Your Office Visit

When you visit your healthcare provider, he or she will ask you about your symptoms, do a physical examination, and may order medical tests. All of this ensures an accurate diagnosis.

But just what is a diagnosis? It is a word used so often that many people underestimate how important it is to the proper treatment of a disease. At its simplest, diagnosis is a determination of the problem so that a treatment plan can be devised. But with complex diseases like arthritis, where there are many options for treatment, diagnosis is even more important.

If disease is, as some have described it, a journey to a foreign land, then diagnosis tells you what land it is and provides the best road map for making it through safely. Diagnosis is as much an art as it is a science, as much intuition as it is a review of objective facts. Several elements are needed to reach a diagnosis.

The Medical History

Although the word "history" conjures up images of past events, a medical history is really an accounting of what has happened that prompted you to see a healthcare provider. Many health professionals rely more on the medical history than anything else to determine whether or not you have arthritis. They will then use the physical examination and medical tests to either narrow the possibilities of diagnosis or better refine it. The more information you can give your healthcare provider and the more clearly you can articulate or document it, the better the chances that you will receive an accurate diagnosis.

While taking the medical history, your healthcare provider will ask about symptoms such as pain and stiffness, when the symptoms started, how long they lasted, and how the condition has interfered with daily activities. For instance, has it affected the way you walk or get dressed in the morning? Can you still climb stairs or open doors?

It is important to know that while most people with arthritis feel pain, not everyone experiencing pain has arthritis. In particular, pain that is bad enough to awaken you from sleep at night could be a sign of soft tissue inflammation, as is the case with bursitis or tendinitis. Or it could be a sign of significant joint damage, a bone fracture, or even nerve entrapment. If pain awakens you at night, mention it during your office visit.

Your healthcare provider will also ask whether any of your immediate family members have had arthritis and, if so, what type. And he or she will ask about some issues you may consider irrelevant but that could be pertinent, such as medications you are taking and whether you have any allergies.

That's a lot to remember. Most people can't recall all the details. To make it easier on yourself and to communicate better with your healthcare provider, you may want to begin charting your symptoms as soon as you begin to notice them. You can use the sample chart located in Table 1 and bring it with you during your initial diagnostic workup. Your healthcare provider may ask you the following questions (adapted from a booklet by The Arthritis Foundation) to determine if you have arthritis:

1. Where does it hurt?
2. When does it hurt? In the morning? After exercise?
3. When did it start to hurt?
4. Has the pain been constant or does it come and go?
5. Is the area swollen?
6. What daily tasks are you having trouble with?
7. Have you ever injured the joint in some way?
8. Do you have a job or a hobby that involves repetitive motions?
9. Has anyone in your family ever had arthritis?
10. Has anyone in your family ever had similar symptoms?

The Physical Examination

Your healthcare provider may first do a basic medical examination, listening to your heart and lungs, and examining your joints for any signs of swelling and/or inflammation. He or she will then press your joints gently to determine if there is any tenderness in the area and may also gently move or stretch the affected joints to see whether your range of motion (or ability to move them) is limited in any way.

Table 1. **Symptom Tracking Chart**

Pain

Where does it hurt? (*Circle*)

Back

Elbows   *One or both?*

Feet   *One or both?*

    Ankles

    Ball of foot

    Toes

Hand   *One or both?*

    Fingers

    Thumbs

    Wrist

Hip   *One side or both?*

Jaw   *One side or both?*

Knees   *One side or both?*

Neck

Shoulders   *One or both?*

Other places *(specify)*:

When does it hurt?

Morning or upon waking
Afternoon, after activity
Evening or while in bed

If you have pain when you get up in
the morning, how long is it until
you feel more limber? How many
minutes or hours?

_____

Is the pain constant? Or does it
occur a few times a day or a few
times a week?

_____

Give details, such as what you are
doing when you notice the pain:

_____

When did you first notice the pain?

Date, as best you can remember:

_____

Were you injured or ill right before
the pain started?

_____

How much pain have you experienced
in the past week?

No pain
Moderate pain
Severe pain

Impact on Daily Activities

What types of activities do you have
trouble doing?

Opening jars
Opening a door
Turning the key in the car's ignition
Getting dressed in the morning
Going up or down stairs

How far can you walk on level ground
without experiencing pain?

_____

Do you have to lean back to put on
your shoes or socks?

_____

Can you get off the toilet seat
without difficulty?

_____

Do you walk with a limp?

_____

Can you drive a car?

_____

Does the pain awaken you from
sleep at night?

_____

What makes the pain better?

_____

What makes it worse?

_____

Other Symptoms

Is there any swelling around the
affected joint?

Yes
No
There was swelling, but it
disappeared

(*continued on following page*)

Table 1. **Symptom Tracking Chart** *(continued)*

Have you had any stomach trouble or flu-like symptoms that won't go away?	Yes *If so, please describe.* No
Have you felt unusually tired recently? Do you find you lose energy in the course of the day?	Yes *If so, please describe.* No

Past Injuries or Illness

Have you ever injured the affected joint?	Yes *If so, when, where, and how?* No
Have you ever done physically demanding work, especially tasks that involve repeated movements of certain joints?	Yes *If so, describe work and duration.* No
What type of sports do you play or hobbies do you have? Do you exercise regularly? Provide as much information as possible.	_____ _____
Have you ever had an operation?	Yes *If so, when and what type?* No
What major illnesses have you had in the past?	_____
What medications are you currently taking? *Please list all.*	_____
Are you allergic to any medications? *Please list all.*	_____
Has anyone in your immediate family ever had arthritis (parents, grandparents, siblings)?	_____

The physical examination helps narrow the possibilities for an initial diagnosis that your healthcare provider has developed after taking down your medical history. The physical examination is used to rule out some possibilities or to better define the type, location, and severity.

Medical Tests

The type of medical tests ordered by your healthcare provider will depend on the type of symptoms you have described. If osteoarthritis is suspected, your healthcare provider may ask a radiologist to take an X ray of the affected joint. Or a blood sample may be ordered to determine if you are a candidate for treatment with NSAIDs, nonsteroidal anti-inflammatory drugs (discussed in greater detail in chapter 5). If there is swelling in the area or if the diagnosis is in question, the joint fluid may also be removed for diagnostic purposes. Further details about the type of medical tests ordered when osteoarthritis is suspected are contained in chapter 6.

If your healthcare provider suspects rheumatoid arthritis or some other type of arthritis, he or she will likely order a blood test to detect any telltale antibodies or signs of inflammation. In some cases your healthcare provider may also order an X ray of the affected joint to determine the extent of damage, and may withdraw synovial fluid from your joint to determine if your arthritis has been caused by inflammation, such as rheumatoid arthritis, an infection, or a crystal disease such as gout. More details on the types of medical tests conducted if rheumatoid arthritis is suspected are included in chapter 7.

Treatment Recommendations

Your healthcare provider will develop a diagnosis and tell you what kind of arthritis you have and how severe it is. Then you and your healthcare provider will agree on a treatment plan.

Although treatment will vary depending on the type of arthritis you have, most arthritis management strategies involve the following components:

Patient education. Your healthcare provider may give you brochures about the type of arthritis you have or recommend books. If not, ask for any educational materials that are appropriate to your situation. You may also want to ask about any support groups in your area. The Arthritis Foundation, which has local chapters across the country, is especially helpful. These groups may have even more information and will provide emotional support if you need it. The more you learn about the type of arthritis you have, the more you will be able to manage your disease. An educated patient is an empowered patient! (For a list of national organizations that can provide more information about arthritis, see Appendix A.)

Physical and occupational therapy. Depending on the severity of your condition, your healthcare provider may also refer you to a physical or occupational therapist. Typically this is done if you are having trouble walking or getting out of a chair, or experiencing some other disturbance in the way you move.

Physical and occupational therapists evaluate muscle strength, joint stability, and your ability to move. They advise about exercise programs appropriate for you and may also recommend that you obtain assistive devices such as special inserts for your shoes, canes, or walkers. Occupational therapists tend to focus on the joints in the hands and the arms since we use these most often while doing tasks. But there is a lot of overlap between the two professions. More details about physical and occupational therapy will be provided in chapter 10.

Exercise. Whether or not you see a physical therapist, you may be advised to start exercising. Although a workout may be the last thing you want to do if your joints hurt, studies have shown that regular and appropriate exercise improves the health of people with arthritis. If you are not exercising at the time you are diagnosed with arthritis, your healthcare provider or physical therapist will likely recommend that you start. A good exercise program includes *range-of-motion exercises,* which improve flexibility; *strengthening exercises* for the muscles surrounding the affected area, so that they can better support your joints; and *endurance exercises,* such as walking and swimming, to improve cardiovascular health. For more information see chapter 3.

Pain relief. Your healthcare provider will advise you about how to relieve the pain of arthritis. This might include tips about relaxation techniques, since tension can intensify pain, as well as medications. Typical medications include over-the-counter pain relievers such as *Advil* or *Tylenol.* For more severe cases of arthritis, your healthcare provider may recommend a prescription medication such as *non-steroidal anti-inflammatory drugs,* NSAIDs, which reduce pain and, at higher doses, inflammation. (This category includes the new COX-2 inhibitors, which cause fewer stomach ulcers than NSAIDs. See chapter 5 for information about NSAIDs, COX-2 inhibitors, and pain relief.)

Since pain is such a complex phenomenon, many people also find complementary therapies helpful. Ask your healthcare provider about such therapies if you are interested. Further details about complementary medicines are included in chapter 11.

Surgery. If you have an advanced case of arthritis and other strategies are either not appropriate or have not worked, your healthcare provider may recommend surgery. Joint replacement is probably the best known type of surgery for arthritis, but new procedures are being developed that offer other options.

How Treatment Recommendations Are Developed

There is no "one size fits all" when it comes to the treatment of disease, and that is especially true of arthritis. Typically your healthcare provider will recommend an initial therapeutic strategy, discuss the risks and benefits with you, and come to a mutual agreement with you about what steps to take next. You will both monitor the response and whether you are comfortable with the results.

The specific treatment plan you and your healthcare provider decide on may depend on your age, gender, severity and type of arthritis, and past medical history. You must also weigh more subjective factors such as your lifestyle, your own comfort with risk, your view of medications and complementary therapies, and the "price" (both in terms of actual cost and possible side effects) that you are willing to pay to achieve decreased pain and increased function.

The initial strategy may be revised as time goes on, depending on how you respond and how the disease progresses. You may not even need prescription medicine and may respond well to an exercise plan and supportive devices such as splints. Or your pain and other symptoms may be so bad that you need medication. But how you respond to a particular drug is different from how someone else will respond. Treatment plans are seldom static; they often require adjustments.

Many of the treatment strategies discussed in this book have been developed by the American College of Rheumatology. This is the professional nonprofit organization, based in Atlanta, for rheumatologists and associated health professionals in the United States. The American College of Rheumatology develops its treatment guidelines after extensive review and comment by its member rheumatologists and allied health professionals. These guidelines are revised periodically on the basis of new medical information or scientific discoveries or the results of clinical trials, which rigorously test promising new treatments to determine how effective they are.

Clinical Trials: Pioneering Efforts and Proof for the Skeptical

Is a treatment safe? How do you know if it works? And what on earth is a clinical trial anyway? Simply put, clinical trials are the way healthcare providers test new treatments in people and how the federal government decides whether they are safe and effective. Clinical trials may be one of the best kept secrets in medicine. Although the General Accounting Office estimates that as many as twenty thousand clinical trials take place in the United States each year, many Americans have never heard of them.

For healthcare providers, clinical trials offer evidence as to whether a given medication or medical device actually benefits patients. Participating in a clinical trial offers people the chance to try treatments not yet available to the general public. These trials take place only after laboratory studies have shown that the new treatment has potential. Some clinical trials involve new types of medications; others involve new combinations of drugs—to see if they are more effective when used together rather than one at a time. Still other clinical trials test the safety and effectiveness of new medical devices. Recently, some complementary and alternative treatments, such as acupuncture, have also been studied because of strong anecdotal evidence that they may be effective.

Why Clinical Trials Are Conducted

The federal Food and Drug Administration (FDA) is charged with guarding the public's safety when it comes to food, cosmetics, and new drugs and medical devices. Before any new medication or device can be marketed, it must first win FDA approval, and the FDA bases its decisions on the results of clinical trials.

You cannot judge the effectiveness of a treatment only on the basis of FDA approval, however. For one thing, some of the most common and acceptable uses of a new medication are discovered after FDA approval (see "off-label" uses on page 71). For another, the FDA regulates vitamins, minerals, and herbs as "dietary supplements" rather than as drugs—and does not require proof of their effectiveness through clinical trials.

FDA Jurisdiction

The Food and Drug Administration must approve the following new treatments before they can be marketed:

- New drugs or medications
- New combinations of drugs
- New medical devices

FDA regulation of the following items, sometimes marketed as "new treatments" for illness, is different from its regulation of drugs and devices:

- Vitamins
- Herbal remedies
- Nutritional supplements

These items are considered nutritional supplements. The FDA oversees their safety, manufacture, and product labeling, but its premarket review is much less stringent than that for new drugs and devices.

Federal regulations aside, the medical community values clinical trials for the information they provide. Medical professionals do not know if a new treatment truly works until it has been tested on enough people to provide a representative sampling of the population with the illness. A treatment that works in one person is considered *anecdotal* evidence of its effectiveness, which is not enough to convince doctors that it will work for their patients.

This is because of something called the *placebo effect*. A placebo is a harmless but ineffectual substance that should have no medical effect—the proverbial "sugar pill." Yet one of the best-documented mysteries in medicine is the placebo effect: If you believe that a new treatment or substance will work, it often does have some beneficial effect even if the substance has no medicinal qualities. Studies since the mid-1950s have found that the placebo effect is responsible for anywhere from 33 to 70 percent of the improvement that patients experienced from a given treatment.

There are many theories about why the placebo effect exists. Some attribute it to the power of positive thinking. Others theorize that our expectation of success inclines us to see improvement even when none exists. Still others think the brain triggers a biological response, unleashing immune system cells and endorphins that reduce pain so that we not only unconsciously will ourselves to get better but actually feel better.

Whatever the reason, healthcare providers need to account for the placebo effect and their own biases when evaluating a new treatment. For this reason, clinical trials are designed according to the most rigorous scientific standards.

The Long Road from Bench to Bedside

When a new treatment is announced in the media, often the only thing that is new about it is the announcement. A new medication can take years to develop and refine before the FDA deems it acceptable for widespread use.

The road from an initial laboratory discovery to an FDA-approved treatment—or from "bench to bedside"—is a long and

Typical Timeline for Drug Development

Years	Task
2–10	Research and development in the laboratory
4	Preclinical testing in the laboratory and in animals
1	Phase 1 trials in people *(safety)*
2	Phase 2 trials in people *(dose, effectiveness)*
3	Phase 3 trials in people *(risks and benefits, comparison with standard therapy)*
12 to 20 years	Total

tortuous one. It can take anywhere from twelve to twenty years from start to finish. The journey takes place in a series of phases.

Preclinical Phase. The process begins when a biotechnology company, medical research center, or pharmaceutical company discovers in laboratory experiments that a compound is promising. This phase is also known as *in vitro* testing.

If the test-tube experiments continue to show promise, the therapy moves into the laboratory animal phase so that scientists can study the treatment *in vivo,* or in a living animal. At this point the scientists also test different doses of the drug to discover if it has any toxic effects that would not be seen in the laboratory.

Phase One. If the animal experiments go well, the drug sponsor asks the FDA for permission to begin testing on people. The number of people who participate in phase one trials is small, perhaps twenty to eighty patients in the entire country, and are generally those who have not responded well to any other treatment.

The primary goal of a phase one study is to determine whether the new medication is safe in people. Researchers also look at how the drug is metabolized by the patient and whether it causes any side effects.

A phase one clinical trial typically takes several months. Seven out of ten medications investigated in a phase one study go on to the next phase.

Phase Two. These also involve a relatively small group of patients, perhaps one hundred to three hundred nationally. In this phase the goal is to determine the proper dose of the medication and whether it is effective.

Typically, phase two studies compare the outcomes of patients who took the medication and those who took a placebo or an already approved drug.

A phase two study typically lasts from several months to several years. Only one-third of the drugs that begin phase two testing go on to the next phase.

Phase Three. These trials involve much larger groups of patients, anywhere from several hundred to several thousand nationally. Phase three trials typically take place simultaneously at multiple research sites across the country.

At this point the new treatment has been deemed reasonably safe and effective. The goal of this large-scale testing is to provide a better understanding of the medication's benefits and risks, side effects, and whether it is more effective than standard therapy.

FDA Approval. The FDA reviews clinical trials as they progress from one phase to another. Approval for marketing is generally considered after phase three testing has concluded.

On rare occasions the FDA or the research institution conducting the study may halt a trial before its scheduled completion. If patients enrolled in the study suffer serious adverse reactions to the experimental medication, the trial will be halted for safety reasons. It is also possible, if the benefits of the new treatment are overwhelming, that the research institution will decide to halt the trial so that the new medication can be submitted to the FDA for expedited approval.

Once the FDA approves a particular medication, it issues a set of guidelines on the approved use of the new drug. This is usually very narrowly focused—for example, approving rofecoxib *(Vioxx),* one of the new COX-2 inhibitors, only for use by those with osteoarthritis or acute pain. But the medication may also be effective for other forms of arthritis and other types of pain.

Every medication marketed in the United States includes a package insert (typically written in small print because it is so lengthy) detailing which illnesses it can be used to treat and the doses that are appropriate. It also involves a listing of *indications,* or conditions where the medication is appropriate, and *contraindications,* where the medication is not appropriate, and when treatment should be stopped.

Phase Four: Testing and "Off-Label" Uses. Phase four testing takes place after FDA approval, often even after the drug has reached the market. This phase can be formal or informal. Formal testing is for long-term effectiveness, side effects, and cost effectiveness compared with standard therapy.

Off-label uses are those not specified in the FDA package insert. The FDA does not prevent doctors from prescribing the medication for uses other than those specified. New uses for approved medications are generally revealed gradually through the experiences of individual healthcare providers and in reports shared in medical journals.

Once again, the important thing to remember is to ask your healthcare provider if a newly approved drug is appropriate for your situation. He or she is familiar with what is being reported at medical conferences and in medical journals, and will be able to make a recommendation.

Participating in a Clinical Trial

Whatever the purpose of a clinical trial, if you enroll in one, you become a pioneer of sorts. You are venturing into the unknown and helping to map the terrain.

Clinical trials are open to children as well as adults and take place in a variety of medical settings: hospitals, private medical offices, and community clinics. You may decide to participate in a clinical trial because it gives you access to a new medication not otherwise available for several years. Or you may be put off by the terms *investigational* and *experimental.* Clinical trials require you to make decisions and choices that can be complicated. They have benefits and risks. They offer promises and pitfalls. It is best to approach them with an open mind and healthy skepticism.

Factors to Consider When Deciding About a Clinical Trial

Clinical trials are not for everyone. On the plus side:

- The clinical trials are monitored closely by healthcare providers, so you will be assured quality care.
- The treatment being evaluated may turn out to be better than the standard treatments currently available.
- Because clinical trials test new treatments, you will be one of the first to benefit if the treatment is an improvement over current therapy.
- Your participation will help advance medical knowledge, so you may help other patients.

But there are also risks involved:

- The new medication or device being evaluated may turn out to be no more effective than standard therapy.
- Participants in most clinical trials are assigned at random to the new treatment or to standard therapy or placebo. You are not able to choose which treatment you receive.
- Especially in early phase clinical trials, the risks and side effects of the new therapy may not be known.
- Your health insurance plan may not cover the costs of participating in a clinical trial because the treatment is considered experimental. In most clinical studies the costs involved—including medications, checkups, and laboratory tests required—are covered by the research project itself or by the institution conducting the study. You should inquire.

Because the decision about whether to participate is a complicated one, it is best to talk it over carefully with your doctor.

Questions to Ask Your Healthcare Provider

Before deciding whether to participate in a clinical trial, you should be certain that you understand as much as you can about the new treatment, its risks, and its benefits. Here are questions to ask:

1. What does the new treatment involve?
2. How does it differ from the type of treatment I would receive if I didn't take part in this clinical trial?
3. What is the purpose of this clinical trial? What is it trying to determine?
4. Is this the first time this treatment has been tested in people (that is, is it a phase one trial)?
5. If it has been tested on other people, how many? What were the results?
6. What phase of testing am I participating in?
7. What are the benefits of participating?
8. What are the risks?
9. When will I know if this treatment is working? How will I know?
10. What type of tests will I have to undergo while participating?
11. What side effects should I expect from this treatment? How long will they last?
12. Where will treatment take place?
13. How long will it last?
14. If I have any concerns about the clinical trial, whom should I call? Is someone available seven days a week, twenty-four hours a day if I need to talk?
15. Will my health insurance plan cover this clinical trial?
16. What steps are you taking to ensure my privacy?

Above All, Become Your Own Advocate

As you sort through treatment options, remember that you are your own best advocate. The reality of managed care is that many health-care providers have much less time to simply talk nowadays. Their time with you may be limited. The more you can do to prepare for your office visits, using the information given in this chapter, the more productive those visits will be.

You are also your own best advocate outside of the medical setting. Some well-meaning friend may tell you about an arthritis treatment that worked for someone he or she knew. Or you'll see an advertisement in a newspaper or magazine that touts the benefits of a medication you've never heard about. Or you'll subscribe to an

---

Sorting Hope from Hype on New Arthritis Treatments

Words to be wary of:

Cure: There is currently no cure for arthritis. If you see "arthritis" and "cure" in the same sentence, read the fine print. It is likely there will be some disclaimer.

Medical miracle: There are few medical miracles in this world. And certainly complex diseases such as arthritis have several causes and will require multiple treatment strategies.

Has no side effects: Almost every medication has side effects. The real issue is the type of side effects and how severe they are.

Clinically proven: Does this mean the treatment was tested in rigorous clinical trials? Or does it mean one healthcare provider working in some type of medical setting has seen some results?

Doctors recommend: Which doctors? Does a professional society like the American College of Rheumatology recommend the treatment or just a few individual doctors?

Questions to ask yourself when you hear about a new treatment:

1. What is the source of the information? (Healthcare provider? Medical story in a professional or peer-reviewed journal? Medical story in a newspaper? Advertisement? Internet? Good friend or coworker?)
2. How reliable is the source? Does the source have any healthcare training?
3. What evidence is presented to support the treatment's effectiveness? How many people have benefited? What is the scientific basis, or logic, for the treatment?
4. Have any adverse side effects been discussed? If so, how severe are they?
5. Has the FDA approved the treatment?
6. How long does it take to experience benefits from the new treatment?
7. How much does it cost? Is the cost reimbursable through your health insurance plan?

Internet news service about arthritis and receive periodic updates on new treatments or studies.

While there is no way to anticipate every bit of information you may be exposed to, it would be helpful to create a list that includes questions to ask yourself—or the source of the new information—in order to make an initial judgment about whether the new treatment is really effective or just hype. This is one more way to ensure that when you call your healthcare provider to seek his or her advice, you will be that much more informed.

CHAPTER 5

Treating Pain and Inflammation

Joan had coped with a lot in her life, and so she took the pain of arthritis in stride, at least in the beginning. She first noticed the pain about five years ago. Her knees and back were stiff when she got out of bed in the morning, but by lunchtime she felt better and could move more easily. Her healthcare provider recommended a mild pain reliever, and that worked well for a while.

But in the past year the pain had worsened considerably. It was getting so bad that she could no longer play with her grandchildren when they came to visit and certainly couldn't lift them into the air the way her husband could. Joan couldn't garden as well as she used to; her back and shoulders became too stiff. But now the weeds were taking over the yard, and she was beginning to feel tired and fatigued and just plain overwhelmed.

To make matters worse, her healthcare provider had retired. Her new healthcare provider, whom she didn't know well, wanted her to switch medications, but she wasn't sure the side effects would be worth it. As for her husband, he thought it was all in her head. Sometimes she thought it was, too.

IT HURTS. That pretty much sums up the most common complaint about arthritis. It hurts a lot. For some people the pain is constant. For others it ebbs and flows. It is worse in the morning or wakes you at night. Take your pick. And the real question is: What can you do to make it go away?

People with certain types of arthritis will also suffer from inflammation. The joint becomes swollen, red, and warm to the touch. It will also become stiff as the inflamed tissues interfere with movement. Not only will you be in pain, but you'll also be hobbled. And once again the question will be: What can I do to make it go away?

Fortunately, you have many options to take control of both pain and inflammation. Some you can do on your own; for others you will need to consult with your healthcare provider. Either way, you can do something to alleviate pain and inflammation.

What Is Pain?

Pain is a phenomenon that just about everyone has felt at one time or another, but only recently have doctors and scientists begun to understand the complex process that causes you to say "ouch"—or worse. We know enough to provide a sort of aerial view of the process, mapping out a terrain that includes the brain, a network of nerves throughout the body, sensitive nerve endings, and multiple chemicals unleashed by the immune system whenever you suffer an injury. But the close-up shots that provide even more helpful information are only now being developed. What kind of chemicals are involved in pain transmission, and exactly how does the brain interpret these signals?

We know this much: Pain normally functions as a sentry, alerting you to danger and prompting you to do something to protect yourself. Although often feared and disliked by anyone who has suffered it, pain is actually one of our best defenses against serious injury. Pain is the body's alert that something needs to be avoided or fixed.

Anyone who has touched a hot burner by mistake knows that "ouch" is followed by an instinctive pulling away, and that reflex action is so quick that it probably feels instantaneous rather than a two-step process. Treat the burn, and the pain will subside after a while.

Pain May Be Different for Men and Women

Recent research has shown that although we all share common pain pathways, we perceive pain in very different ways. For one thing, men and women appear to differ in how they experience pain and how they respond to pain relievers. One group of researchers reported that one medication used to relieve dental pain (nalbuphine) is more effective for women than men and at some doses may even worsen the pain for men. Another team has reported that ibuprofen, an NSAID commonly used to treat arthritis, is more effective in men than in women. This team also reported that women's response to ibuprofen seems to depend on the point in their menstrual cycles it is taken. These observations about potential differences in response between men and women raise interesting questions, but further study about how gender affects response to pain relief is needed.

Pain May Play a Part in Healing

Pain may also function as more than just your body's alert system; some think it actually plays an important part in the healing process. According to this theory, once inflammation—the body's response to injury—reaches a certain critical point, you will feel pain. And the chemicals involved in creating that painful sensation somehow also subdue inflammation before it continues unabated, causing more harm than good.

In most forms of arthritis, the pain does not subside but continues long after its usefulness is over. "Alert. Danger. Something is wrong," your knee is screaming through the pain. And even if you do something—rest the joint, take a pain medication—the pain may still be there waiting for you once the drugs wear off.

The Role of Endorphins

Fortunately, there is hope. Over the years researchers have learned more about the dynamics of pain and how to treat it. One of the more intriguing findings is that the body produces its own pain control substances known as endorphins. These chemicals actually block pain signals, much as medications do. The challenge is in learning how to activate them. Some people find that simple techniques such as a massage or applying a hot compress to an affected joint lessens the pain, perhaps because endorphins are released.

Pain operates on several levels at once—physical, mental, and emotional—and therefore treatment strategies also tend to be multifaceted. The basic components of a pain management plan are outlined in the pages that follow. Talk with your own healthcare provider about these options and find the combination that works best for you.

What Is Inflammation?

Many types of arthritis also involve inflammation, which is a specific type of immune system response.

Inflammation begins when a joint is injured in some way. Perhaps you have an accident, ranging from something simple, twisting your ankle, to something complex, like the bone-jarring impact of an automobile collision. Or you may have been exposed to a bacterial infection, as in the case of Lyme disease. Perhaps the cause of the injury is not known.

Whatever the cause, once the joint is injured, the immune system responds with inflammation. Blood vessels widen, or dilate, and blood and other fluids seep into the affected area. This increased blood flow allows rescue worker cells to travel quickly to the site of the injury. As blood flows into the tissue surrounding the injury, the area becomes inflamed. You will likely feel pain and warmth, and see the injured area swell up.

If you have ever banged a knee and felt the resulting pain, stiffness, and warmth in the area, you have some idea of the type of inflammation that occurs in arthritis. The difference is that, with some types of arthritis, the inflammation does not subside. For any one of a number of reasons, your well-intentioned immune system begins hurting your joint rather than helping it. Eventually the process of inflammation may further damage bones and the joint structures, compounding the problem. (For a more detailed explanation of how the immune system and the process of inflammation can damage joints, see chapter 2.)

Because pain and inflammation are often the most vexing symptoms of arthritis, we will explore both in greater detail in the pages that follow, and you will learn how to cope with and treat them.

Why We Feel Pain

Pain is really a form of communication. In verbal communication, one person speaks, you hear the sounds with your ears, and then your brain interprets the sounds as words. Similarly, certain chemicals at the site of an injury send signals, which are then "heard" by nerve endings located close by and interpreted in your brain as pain.

The nerve endings have special receptors known as nociceptors that receive sensory information (touch, heat, cold, and the like) and in turn send a signal to the brain for interpretation. The sensory information is interpreted as pain when the communication becomes physically unpleasant and emotionally distressing—anything from mild discomfort to eye-popping, teeth-grinding agony.

Nociceptors vary according to their location in your body and the type of information they communicate to your brain. Many are located near the surface of your skin. Some are extremely sensitive and communicate everything from warmth to firm pressure. Other nerves react only to dramatic sensations such as burns and cuts. Other parts of your body, notably tendons and blood vessels, have different types of nociceptors.

Nociceptors also respond to certain chemicals produced by your immune system. In an arthritic joint, for instance, an enzyme known as cyclooxygenase (COX) gives rise to other chemicals known as prostaglandins. Once nociceptors in the area detect prostaglandins, a pain signal is sent to your brain. Recent research is uncovering other chemicals, such as one known as substance P, that also appear to send pain signals to the brain. Undoubtedly others will be discovered.

Why Arthritis Causes Pain

Not everyone who has arthritis experiences pain, but for those who do, there can be many reasons for it.

- Damage to the joints: As the cartilage wears down and the space between the bones grows smaller, all the components of your joints (bones, surrounding tissues, and muscles) are less cushioned against the impact of any movement. In addition, bits of the cartilage may break off as fragments, or bone spurs that develop may put pressure on your nerves or other sensitive tissues.
- Muscle strain: As the muscles and ligaments surrounding the affected joint are required to work harder in order to protect the area against the jolt of movements, they become strained. You may begin to feel pain as a result.
- Fatigue: As the disease progresses, your body grows tired from the assault on the joints. Fatigue is part of any serious disease process and can make you more susceptible to feeling pain.
- Inflammation: Inflammation does not affect everyone with arthritis. (People with osteoarthritis, for instance, may never experience inflammation.) But when inflammation does occur and continues for too long, it places more strain on your joints. The process of inflammation may also exacerbate the pain because chemicals at the site of the inflamed joint send pain signals to the brain, adding to whatever discomfort you are already feeling.

Pain from arthritis might occur after you have exercised too much or after you have spent the afternoon in a chair and not exercised at all. Some people feel pain when they first get up in the morning; others begin to ache at the end of the day.

Arthritis pain varies in intensity from person to person, owing to differences in the severity of joint damage. People also differ in their pain thresholds, the point at which they perceive pain. Part of the reason may be physical, having to do with normal variations in nerve sensitivity. But there is also a psychological component to pain that can make the experience worse or better depending on the emotion. Pain often causes anxiety (Is the disease getting worse? Won't this ever end?) that will worsen the sensation. Chronic pain can lead to depression, which in turn can lower your ability to cope with the pain and will make it seem worse.

Pain Cycles

The Arthritis Foundation refers to a "pain cycle": Negative emotional factors can affect the perception of pain and limit your physical abilities. Pain that causes depression may result in your getting out less and less. Your overall physical conditioning then deteriorates, your movements become even more restricted and your joints stiffer, and more pain results, leading to an even deeper depression.

Fortunately, it is possible to break this cycle. The approach combines outside interventions such as medication and internal adjustments in thinking. Put simply, your healthcare provider may prescribe a medication and ask that you take it with a glass that is half full rather than half empty. This is not just happy talk. Study after study has shown that people with arthritis pain who learn to deal with it in a positive way actually end up feeling less pain and suffering less disability than people who dwell on their aches and become depressed.

Rheumatology researchers have also reported that people who participate in self-management programs, such as the one offered by The Arthritis Foundation, experience less joint pain and make fewer visits to healthcare providers while enjoying more physical activity and overall well-being. The positive feelings created by being more in control of the situation appear to dampen the perception of pain. That is why we want to help you empower yourself.

How Pain and Inflammation Are Diagnosed

It is relatively easy for your healthcare provider to determine if you are suffering from inflammation. Just looking at your joint will provide some clues: If the area is red, swollen, and warm to the touch, it is showing the classic signs of inflammation. To confirm the diagnosis, your healthcare provider may order a blood test, which can be analyzed for the telltale chemicals involved in inflammation.

TABLE 2. Communicating Pain and Health Status

In some cases a picture can be worth a thousand words. Your healthcare provider may ask you to *show* how much it hurts or how much your health has been affected by using a visual guide similar to the one below.

How much pain have you had because of your condition in the past week? Place a mark on the line below to indicate how severe your pain has been:

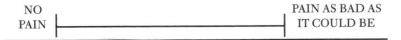

```
NO                                                PAIN AS BAD AS
PAIN  |————————————————————————————————|   IT COULD BE
```

Pain is not as easy to diagnose. One of the vexing things about pain is that it is an extremely personal phenomenon; no one else can "feel" your pain but you even when it affects you like an earthquake, shaking you to your core. While there are pain scales that can help others understand just how much it hurts, there are no objective tests that can graph the tremors of your very real pain.

Because pain is such a personal and subjective experience, it needs to be communicated as clearly as possible to your healthcare provider. It's hard for most people to remember when something hurt and exactly how long it hurt. You may therefore want to use a pain chart to keep track of your symptoms day by day. (You can use the Symptom Tracking Chart in chapter 4 as a starting point or the visual pain scale above.)

It is also good to start developing a vocabulary of pain that will enhance your ability to communicate what exactly you are feeling. "It hurts" is vague. "It aches [or throbs or burns]" is more specific and will help your healthcare provider advise about treatment.

To determine how much pain you are suffering and what may be causing it, your healthcare provider may do any of the following:

- Take your medical history, asking when the pain started, where it is located, how much it hurts, whether it is constant or if it comes and goes, and what makes it worse and what makes it better.
- Ask what medications you are currently taking or have taken in the past, at what doses, and whether they are providing pain relief.
- Do a physical examination.
- Take blood or urine samples for analysis in the laboratory; this will help determine what type of arthritis you have.
- Ask that you undergo additional tests such as X rays, CAT scans, or MRI, which will produce images of bones, cartilage, tendons, ligaments, and other structures beneath the skin. These will help your provider better understand what the joint looks like and what may be causing the pain.
- Conduct studies to determine which nerves are affected. This is done by inserting needles beneath the skin to numb particular nerves, much as your dentist does with Novocain.

The medical history, medication review, and physical exam are effective in defining the type of pain you have and how it should be treated. Your healthcare provider may take additional steps if he or she needs more information.

How Pain and Inflammation Are Treated

There is no "magic pill" that can make the pain go away. When healthcare providers talk about a pain management plan, they emphasize your role as a manager. Pain has to be managed as much as it has to be treated. That means you, the person affected by the pain, will fare best if you take an active role in dealing with it. You can't change the pain, but you can change how you react to it.

Typically, a pain management strategy involves several components—and perhaps several healthcare providers—at once. Your team might include a physician, rheumatologist (a specialist in diseases involving the bones, joints, and muscles), nurse, physical therapist, psychiatrist, and/or surgeon. Or one healthcare provider might weave various perspectives together. It depends on your circumstances.

Your pain management plan will likely consist of two broad segments: medication and other types of interventions.

The First Step: Education

Everyone knows what arthritis is, right? Wrong. How many people know that the term encompasses more than one hundred different diseases? So the first step is to educate yourself about your joints, about the type of arthritis you have, and about the types of treatments available to you.

Fortunately, you don't have to approach this the way you approached term papers in school. Most likely your healthcare provider will have brochures, videos, and pamphlets on hand to help you familiarize yourself with your condition. A number of helpful organizations can also provide information, either in print form or over the Internet. (See appendix A for a list of organizations.)

Take a Self-Help Course

Some HMOs and organizations such as The Arthritis Foundation offer self-help or self-management courses that you may find
useful. In these courses you learn how to gain more control over
your symptoms. Part of the focus is on changing your attitudes
toward pain and arthritis. Focusing on the positive aspects of your
life rather than on the negative is an effective way to deal with
pain. Dwelling on the pain will not make it better and will only
make you more aware of it. And people who think about their pain
a lot tend to report more pain than people who try not to think of
it. Distract yourself by doing activities you enjoy such as talking on
the phone with a friend or watching a funny movie. Focus on positive emotions.

Self-help courses will also help you change the way you think
and react to stressful situations—no matter what your age. It just
takes a little practice and the desire to try. For instance, stop
saying the glass is half empty and start saying it is half full. Or, in
terms of arthritis, try not to say, "My knee hurts, and I don't want
to go outside and take a walk." Instead say, "My knee will feel
better once I get outside and loosen it up and breathe in some
fresh air."

Finally, self-help courses will offer tips on stress reduction. Stress
and tension are natural reactions to any chronic illness, but they
only heighten sensitivity to pain. To relax, try some deep-breathing
techniques or light an aromatic candle and sit quietly. You could
take a meditation course as well.

Join a Support Group

People who join support groups for their illness tend to do better
than people who do not. There is the practical side: You pick up
self-care tips from other participants. And there is the emotional
side: You get support from people who are going through the same
thing you are.

To find a support group in your area, contact the local chapter of The Arthritis Foundation or check with your HMO or healthcare provider for referrals. Your local newspaper may also list self-help or support groups.

Lose Weight

Losing weight does not sound as if it would ease pain. If anything, the very idea might sound painful. But excess weight places extra pressure on the joints, especially the weight-bearing joints such as the knees and hips. That can worsen both your arthritis and the amount of pain you feel.

Losing weight has several advantages for people with arthritis. It reduces the pressure on joints that are already affected by arthritis. It may prevent or slow the development of osteoarthritis in joints that are not yet affected. And it is good for your overall health and well-being, which in turn makes you better able to cope with the pain of arthritis.

Exercise

Exercise can be the first step in turning a pain cycle into a wellness cycle. That may seem odd. When your joints hurt, it's natural not to want to move. But that will only exacerbate the problem. Joints that are already stiff will only become more difficult to bend if you don't move them. And as discussed in chapter 3, an exercise plan improves your overall health and your ability to cope with the symptoms of arthritis.

Fortunately, many types of exercise are safe to do because they are low impact and won't hurt the joint. These include swimming, walking, and range-of-motion exercises. Be sure to work with your healthcare provider and/or a physical therapist to devise a fitness plan that is safe and beneficial. Start off slow and gradually increase the level of your workouts.

Range-of-motion exercises are regular, gentle, rhythmic movements that can help maintain flexibility. If you are unable to do them on your own, you can benefit from assisted active motion exercises in which another person (a friend or personal trainer) keeps an arthritic joint, such as the wrist, immobile while helping to move another joint, such as the elbow. By stabilizing the arthritic joint, it is easier to move other joints and prevent stiffness from developing in them as well.

Passive range-of-motion exercises, in which someone actually stretches your arthritic joint without any assistance from you, may be used if your joint is very inflamed. It's important to keep your joints moving because lack of motion can lead to stiffening of the joint.

More advanced exercises, such as aerobics and weight training, can also be helpful if you have arthritis—but only when undertaken with the guidance of your healthcare provider or physical therapist.

Aerobic exercises improve your overall well-being by increasing oxygen intake and cardiovascular functioning while strengthening muscles. An aerobics program may include endurance exercises, such as walking, and resistance exercises, in which you build strength by pushing against something.

A water aerobics program actually includes both types of exercises and is probably the best way to begin. The water reduces body weight and decreases strain on joints, yet it provides the resistance that helps to strengthen muscles. Before long, your endurance increases and stamina builds.

You could even undertake weight training. But rather than going from machine to machine at a local health club, you should focus on isolated muscles. Start with small weights and increase repetitions slowly. For instance, your biceps can be strengthened by lifting an 8-ounce bag of sugar, curling your hand toward your shoulder. Repeat the motion five times to start and eventually increase the repetitions to ten curls.

You may wish to avoid some exercises if you have advanced arthritis. One is overhead weight lifting if your shoulder is affected. Some exercises can also make arthritis worse if the disease is advanced and located in the weight-bearing joints, such as the hips.

If you would like to begin exercising, first get a good musculoskeletal evaluation from your healthcare provider, who can advise you about which areas of your body to concentrate on in a fitness program and offer you guidelines to ensure that you don't hurt yourself.

More information about exercises you can do to help your arthritis is presented in chapter 10.

Use Joint Supports and Protective Devices

To ease pressure on the joint, your healthcare provider may recommend that you use a brace or splint. This not only protects your joint, but also lets it rest. A device such as a cane or walker may also help you walk more easily and provide you with the confidence to get out and about without fear of falling. Properly used, these devices can help reduce the pressure on arthritic joints and decrease pain. Special inserts for shoes, such as wedged insoles, can provide additional support and help correct any abnormalities caused by arthritis.

Treating Pain and Inflammation with Medication

While there is no "magic pill" to take away the pain or inflammation of arthritis, there are a number of medications available that can be used in conjunction with other strategies.

Some of the medications discussed below treat pain; others treat both pain and inflammation. Although cost may be the last thing you want to think about when you're in pain, it's wise to do so (and spare yourself a different kind of pain later on). Costs of medications vary widely, and in this era of managed care, your health insurance carrier may pay for all your medication, for part of it, or for none of it. (See Table 3 for more information about costs and health insurance coverage of arthritis drugs.)

TABLE 3. Costs and Health Insurance Coverage of Arthritis Drugs

Sample Costs of Drugs

In the chart below you'll find the average national retail prices and estimated annual costs for some of the most commonly prescribed medications for arthritis.

Drug (Brand Name/ Generic Name)	Standard Dose	Average National Retail Price	Estimated Yearly Cost
Arthrotec	2 tablets/day (75 mg)	$85.86	$1,030.32
Celebrex	1 tablet/day (200 mg)	$72.60	$871.20
Daypro	2 tablets/day (60 mg)	$88.21	$1,058.52
Diclofenac	2 tablets/day (75 mg)	$47.35	$568.20
Ibuprofen	1 tablet/day (800 mg)	$8.34	$100.08
Lodine XL	2 tablets/day (400 mg)	$89.50	$1,074.00
Naproxen	2 tablets/day (500 mg)	$23.47	$281.64
Relafen	2 tablets/day (500 mg)	$73.83	$885.96
Vioxx	1 tablet/day (12.5 mg)	$60.60	$727.20

Data derived from The Arthritis Foundation (*Arthritis Today*, Sept./Oct. 1999, p. 43), based on information from D. P. Hamacher & Associates, Inc., and Merck Co., Inc.

What to Know About Drug Coverage

- Just because a medication has been approved by the FDA does not mean your health plan will cover it. Many managed care plans and even government programs have formularies—a list of drugs they will cover. If your medication is not on the formulary, it may not be covered.
- Your health insurance company may require that you meet certain conditions before the drug is paid for. Sometimes you have to try a

cheaper medication and fail on it before you can receive a more expensive one.

- Some health insurance plans require that you make a co-payment for drugs, and the co-payment may be higher if the drug is not on the company's formulary.
- Your health insurance plan may have an annual limit on the amount it will reimburse you for drug costs.
- Exact terms of your coverage may change from year to year, so read your current policy carefully and call a representative if you don't understand something.
- Medicare generally does not pay for prescription drugs. Some people on Medicare purchase supplemental policies to cover their prescriptions (although co-pays and annual limits may apply).
- Medicaid benefits are determined by state, but generally Medicaid will pay for prescription medications on its approved formulary.

Questions to Ask About Your Health Insurance Coverage

- Is this medication covered in full, in part, or not at all?
- Is there an annual limit to my coverage?
- Are there any requirements I have to fulfill before this medication will be paid for?

As always, it's best to check with your healthcare provider to determine the medications that are most appropriate for you.

Analgesics

Analgesics are medications that relieve pain without reducing inflammation. Analgesics are highly effective at reducing mild or moderate pain, similar to that of a headache or toothache. They do not have the side effects common in other medications such as NSAIDs.

Analgesics work quickly, usually within an hour. The relief from pain generally lasts four to eight hours. These medications work by preventing pain signals from being sent in the first place or by preventing your brain from receiving and interpreting pain impulses.

Acetaminophen, one of the most commonly used analgesics, is the active ingredient in a number of over-the-counter medications, including brand names such as aspirin-free *Anacin, Excedrin,* and *Tylenol.* A list of the most commonly used analgesics is provided in Table 4.

TABLE 4. **Analgesics**

Drug (Generic Name)	Common Brand Names	Standard Dose
Over-the-Counter		
Acetaminophen	*Anacin* (aspirin free)	500–1,000 mg every
	Excedrin caplets	4 to 6 hours as
	Panadol	needed, not to exceed
	Tylenol	4,000 mg/day
Prescription: Narcotic		
Acetaminophen	*Fioricet*	15–60 mg codeine
with codeine	*Phenaphen with*	every 4 hours
	Codeine	as needed
	Tylenol with	
	Codeine	
Propoxyphene	*Darvon, Darvocet*	65 mg every 4 hours
hydrochloride	*PC-Cap*	as needed, not to
	Wygesic	exceed 390 mg/day
Prescription: Non-narcotic		
Tramadol	*Ultram*	50–100 mg every 6
		hours as needed

Data derived from The Arthritis Foundation ("Drug Guide," *Arthritis Today,* Jul./Aug. 1999, p. 34).

Sometimes acetaminophen is combined with other substances, such as caffeine, which might make you jittery and keep you up at night, or antihistamines, which might make you drowsy. We prefer acetaminophen on its own.

When used as directed, acetaminophen does not irritate the stomach as some NSAIDs do, but if you are taking blood-thinning medications such as *Coumadin,* you should ask your healthcare provider whether acetaminophen is right for you. And if you consume three or more alcoholic drinks per day, talk with your healthcare provider before taking aceta-minophen, since this medication can cause liver damage if you drink regularly.

Topical Analgesics

Topical analgesics provide pain relief locally—at a particular joint or joints—rather than systemically. This type of medication is avail-able in creams, lotions, or gels that are spread on the surface of the skin and then penetrate within. If you have mild arthritis pain that is limited to one or two joints or if you want to supplement the effec-tiveness of an oral medication, topical analgesics may be a good option.

A variety of topical analgesics are available in drugstores. Most work in one of three ways. Some distract the nerves with another type of irritant. Known as "counterirritants," these contain ingredi-ents such as menthol, eucalyptus oil, and turpentine oil. Typical brand names are *ArthriCare, Icy Hot,* and *Mineral Ice.* How effec-tive they are is uncertain.

Some topical analgesics relieve pain temporarily by delivering salicylates (the same ingredient in aspirin) through the skin. The topical form appears to inhibit the chemical prostaglandins just as the oral form does and also distracts the nerves through counterirri-tants. Brand names include *Ben-Gay, Mobisyl,* and *Sportscreme.* The effectiveness of these creams is still debated.

The third type of topical analgesic works by countering a chemi-cal known as substance P, a neurotransmitter that appears to trans-mit pain signals to the brain. These creams contain a derivative of a natural ingredient found in cayenne (hot) pepper. As such, they may burn or sting when first used. They are marketed under brand names such as *Capzasin-P* and *Zostrix*.

Topical analgesics are not recommended for use on broken or irritated skin. They also should not be used with a heating pad because it might result in a burn. After applying the creams, make sure to wash your hands before touching your eyes.

Non-steroidal Anti-inflammatory Drugs (NSAIDs)

NSAIDs are among the most frequently prescribed medications in the United States. More than 70 million prescriptions are written annually for them—and that does not include the over-the-counter varieties. With the introduction of COX-2 inhibitors, which provide the benefits of traditional NSAIDs without many of the side effects, the popularity of these drugs is increasing.

TABLE 5. **Non-steroidal Anti-inflammatory Drugs**

Drug (Generic Name)	Common Brand Names	Standard Doses
Short-acting		
Diclofenac potassium	*Cataflam*	**OA°:** 100–150 mg/day **RA°:** 100–200 mg/day
Diclofenac sodium	*Voltaren*	**OA:** 100–200 mg/day **RA:** 150–200 mg/day
Diclofenac sodium with misoprostol	*Arthrotec*	**OA:** 100–150 mg/day **RA:** 100–200 mg/day *Note: These doses apply only to the diclofenac portion; the dosage of misoprostol will vary depending on strength of pill.*
Etodolac	*Lodine* *Lodine XL*	**OA:** 800–1,200 mg/day **RA:** 600–1,200 mg/day
Flurbiprofen	*Ansaid*	200–300 mg/day

Ibuprofen	**Over the Counter:** *Advil* *Motrin IB* *Nuprin*	**Over the Counter:** 200–400 mg/day every 4 to 6 hours; should not exceed 1,200 mg/day
	Prescription: *Motrin*	**Prescription:** 1,200–3,200 mg/day
Ketoprofen	**Over the Counter:** *Actron* *Orudis KT*	**Over the Counter:** 12.5 mg every 4 to 6 hours as needed
	Prescription: *Orudis* *Oruvail*	**Prescription:** 200–225 mg/day 200 mg/day
Meclofenamate sodium	*Meclomen*	200–400 mg/day
Tolmetin sodium	*Tolectin*	1,200 mg/day
Long-acting		
Diflunisal	*Dolobid*	500–1,500 mg/day
Indomethacin	*Indocin*	50–200 mg/day
Nabumetone	*Relafen*	500–1,000 mg/day
Naproxen	*Naprosyn*	500–1,000 mg/day
Naproxen sodium	**Over the Counter:** *Aleve*	220 mg every 8 to 12 hours as needed
	Prescription: *Anaprox*	550–1,100 mg/day
Oxaprozin	*Daypro*	1,200–1,800 mg/day
Piroxicam	*Feldene*	20 mg/day
Sulindac	*Clinoril*	300–400 mg/day
COX-2 Inhibitors		
Celecoxib	*Celebrex*	**OA:** 200 mg/day **RA:** 200–400 mg/day
Rofecoxib	*Vioxx*	**OA:** 12.5 mg–25 mg/day **RA:** Not yet approved

°OA = Dose for osteoarthritis
  RA = Dose for rheumatoid arthritis

Data derived from The Arthritis Foundation ("Drug Guide," *Arthritis Today,* Jul./Aug. 1999, pp. 30–33).

TABLE 6. **Salicylates**

Drug (Generic Name)	Common Brand Names	Standard Dose
Acetylated Salicylates		
Aspirin	*Anacin*	3,600–5,400 mg/day
	Ascriptin	
	Bayer	
	Bufferin	
	Ecotrin	
	Excedrin tablets	
Non-acetylated Salicylates		
Choline magnesium trisalicylate	*CMT*	3,000 mg/day
	Tricosal	
	Trilisate	
Choline salicylate	*Arthropan*	3,480–6,960 mg/day
Magnesium salicylate	*Arthritab*	2,600–4,800 mg/day
	Doan's Pills	
	Magan	
	Mobidin	
Salsalate	*Amigesic*	1,000–3,000 mg/day
	Anaflex 750	
	Disalcid	
	Marthritic	
	Mono-Gesic	
	Salflex	
	Salsitab	
Sodium salicylate	None; available only in generic	3,600–5,400 mg/day

Data derived from The Arthritis Foundation ("Drug Guide," *Arthritis Today,* Jul./Aug. 1999, pp. 32–33).

At low doses, NSAIDs relieve pain; at higher doses they also reduce inflammation. Traditional NSAIDs accomplish this by blocking two enzymes, COX-1 and COX-2. Such *nonselective* NSAIDs include aspirin, ibuprofen (brand names include *Advil* and *Motrin*), and naproxen. COX-2 inhibitors represent a new branch in the NSAID family tree. These medications (*Celebrex* and *Vioxx*) block only the COX-2 enzymes and are therefore considered *selective* NSAIDs.

To some degree aspirin has become the black sheep of the NSAID family. Its benefits are so outweighed by the risks posed that it is not often recommended for the treatment of arthritis. And the COX-2 inhibitors were hailed so extensively by the media that they are in danger of becoming perceived as "goody two-shoes," capable of doing no wrong.

But nothing in medicine is ever that simple. Each of these medications has benefits and risks. (The most commonly recommended NSAIDs are given in Table 5 and Table 6.)

BENEFITS OF NSAIDS

The major benefit is relief of pain, which is your body's way of alerting you to an injury so that you can take steps to avoid further damage. But the process of creating a pain signal in the first place takes several steps. When an injury occurs, the affected tissues produce an enzyme known as cyclooxygenase (COX). This enzyme then helps produce chemicals known as prostaglandins, which initiate the process of inflammation around the site of the injury. Prostaglandins are able to emit a pain signal like an alarm, while at the same time causing blood vessels to dilate. Inflammatory cells race to the scene of the damage. By inhibiting production of COX, NSAIDs prevent this from happening.

Although all NSAIDs share a common mechanism of pain relief, they vary in the amount of time that they remain active—what a physician would call their *half-life*. Short-acting NSAIDs with half-lives ranging from one to eight hours include ibuprofen (*Advil, Motrin*), ketoprofen (*Actron, Orudis*), and flurbiprofen (*Ansaid*). These are taken more often per day.

NSAIDs with a longer half-life (ranging from twelve to twenty-four hours and sometimes longer) include naproxen, piroxicam (*Feldene*), and nabumetone (*Relafen*). These longer-acting agents provide pain relief over a more extended period and may be taken less often.

Thus, while NSAID therapy is common, it is far from simple. Your responsiveness to a certain medication and the type of side effects you experience may differ from someone else's. It is best to work with your healthcare provider to determine whether NSAID treatment is appropriate and, if so, what type of medication and dose to use.

RISKS OF NSAIDs

No medication is risk free. The risk of NSAID side effects appears to relate directly to the amount of medication you take per day and the length of time you take it. Sometimes we also grow more sensitive to the effect of a given drug as we age, possibly because of differences in how we metabolize drugs or because we are taking other medications.

If you should experience side effects, contact your healthcare provider. Sometimes they can be alleviated by taking the NSAID with food or an antacid. Or your healthcare provider may advise you to switch medications.

Gastrointestinal distress: a major risk. Ironically, it is the very ability to block a pain signal that gives NSAIDs such power not only to help but also to hurt. At the center of this paradox is the enzyme briefly described earlier: COX. By inhibiting COX production, NSAIDs solve one problem (pain) but may well cause another (stomach distress).

COX is not one enzyme, as scientists once believed, but two (and new research suggests there could be several versions). COX-1 produces prostaglandins that help maintain the lining of the stomach. COX-2 also produces prostaglandins, but these are primarily involved in sending pain signals and encouraging the process of inflammation. Because traditional NSAIDs block both types of COX enzymes, they relieve pain but may also adversely affect the stomach and kidneys. In fact, the most frequently cited side effect of NSAIDs is mild stomach upset (which affects about 30 to 40 percent of those taking it).

But NSAID use can also lead to more serious problems. These

include the development of *stomach ulcers which can hemorrhage and perforate.* These side effects need to be taken seriously. Researchers have identified others at risk for such complications: those with a history of ulcers, advanced disability, taking higher dosages of NSAIDs and corticosteroids at the same time, and older age groups.

If you experience gastrointestinal distress after taking NSAIDs, your healthcare provider may prescribe a different type of medication or advise you to take something to counteract the side effects, such as H-2 blockers *(Tagamet, Zantac, Pepsid)* and proton-pump inhibitors *(Prilosec* or *Prevacid).* Both types of medication decrease acid production in your stomach. Another type of drug, misoprostol *(Cytotec)* protects your stomach by supplying synthetic versions of prostaglandins.

Less frequent risks. NSAIDs can also cause a number of less common but occasionally serious side effects. These include liver dysfunction, kidney toxicity, rashes and other skin disorders, blood irregularities, and disturbances in the central nervous system.

Like any other drug circulating in the bloodstream, NSAIDs are eventually metabolized in your liver and excreted in urine. On occasion, NSAID use can cause your liver to malfunction, resulting in mild to moderate hepatitis. Generally, this can be reversed when you stop taking whatever NSAID has caused the problem.

Your kidneys filter your blood and rid your body of waste products and excess water by excreting it in urine. Prostaglandins help maintain your kidney's ability to perform these complex tasks. Since NSAID use prevents the production of prostaglandins, these medications may undermine your kidney's functioning. If you have diabetes, hypertension, cardiovascular problems, or a previous history of kidney trouble, you may be at higher risk for developing this complication. Mention these conditions to your healthcare provider if he or she has not asked about them.

If you develop a rash after taking NSAIDs, you may be allergic to the particular medication being used. Your healthcare provider may then prescribe another class of NSAID or recommend a different type of medication altogether.

NSAIDs can lead to the development of ulcers, hemorrhaging, and gastrointestinal perforation. NSAID use may also cause bronchial or lung wheezes. If you have an aspirin allergy, you are particularly at risk for this toxicity.

NSAIDs are able to cross the blood-brain barrier, the protective mechanism that prevents toxins and some medications in your bloodstream from reaching your brain. Because NSAIDs are able to penetrate your brain, they can sometimes disturb the functioning of your central nervous system, resulting in everything from hearing loss and ringing in the ears (tinnitus) to changes in mood and sleep patterns, to confusion and headaches. Generally, these effects will disappear once you stop taking the NSAID that causes them. It is important, however, to notice any such changes and report them to your healthcare provider since ignoring the situation may only make it worse.

Drug interactions. Another risk of NSAID use, as with any medication, is how they interact with other drugs you may be taking or even with food and alcohol. The effect may be different from the effect of the NSAID taken alone.

The impact can be good or bad. In some cases your healthcare provider may prescribe two or more drugs in order to enhance the overall therapeutic value; this approach is known as *combination therapy* and will be discussed in greater detail in chapter 7.

But in other cases, drug interactions can produce harmful effects. For instance, if you are taking blood-thinning medications or anticoagulants such as warfarin, you may be at greater risk for gastrointestinal bleeding. NSAIDs prevent warfarin from binding to certain blood proteins and therefore increase the level of warfarin circulating in your bloodstream.

Be sure to mention any other drugs you may be taking to your healthcare provider so that he or she can determine whether they will interact with a particular NSAID.

Risk Factors for NSAID Side Effects

You are more at risk for developing ulcers if

- You are 65 years or older
- You have had ulcers in the past or have suffered complications from an NSAID
- You are taking multiple NSAIDs at high doses
- You are also receiving corticosteroid therapy

The New Medications

COX-2 Inhibitors

COX-2 inhibitors are medications that can alleviate pain and are thought to have fewer side effects than aspirin or other NSAIDs. This is because they are more specific than NSAIDs and act only on the COX-2 enzyme, which causes pain and inflammation, while ignoring COX-1, which is involved in protecting the lining of the stomach. In doing so, COX-2 inhibitors appear to reduce the most common side effect of NSAIDs: gastrointestinal disorders.

The FDA has approved two COX-2 inhibitors so far: celecoxib, marketed under the brand name *Celebrex*, and rofecoxib, marketed as *Vioxx*. Others are in various stages of development. See Table 5 for information on dosages.

The COX-2 inhibitors were greeted with a great deal of media fanfare and promoted with Madison Avenue hype. In fact, they were dubbed "super aspirins" in the press, not in the laboratory. It is important to remember that these medications have only recently been approved by the FDA and marketed to the public. Clinical studies are under way to determine long-term effectiveness and side effects. A true assessment of the value of the COX-2 inhibitors may not be known for years.

THE SCIENCE BEHIND COX-2 INHIBITORS

COX-2 inhibitors came about only after scientists realized there were at least two forms of an important enzyme known as cyclooxygenase, or COX. COX-1 helps to regulate the kidneys, stomach, and even parts of the vascular system. COX-2, more recently discovered, responds to a particular event such as injury when inflammation and pain result.

But this either/or role for COX-1 and COX-2 is far too simplistic. The more scientists learn about these forms of COX, the more complicated the picture becomes. For instance, some studies show that COX-2 is also found normally in the brain, kidneys, cartilage, and bone even without injury. The main function of COX-1 may be to promote regular functioning of certain tissues, but it also responds to injury in the intestines. The only certainty at this time is that much more has to be learned about each of these enzymes.

Nevertheless, recognizing that COX-2 plays an important role in inflammation and pain, pharmaceutical companies have been developing selective COX-2 inhibitors that do not affect COX-1 function. These medications relieve pain and inflammation but appear to cause less gastrointestinal upset than the older NSAIDs. That is significant. NSAIDs cause about seventy thousand hospitalizations per year for stomach bleeding and other gastrointestinal complications. Worse, they are reported to cause seven thousand deaths per year in the United States.

BENEFITS OF COX-2 INHIBITORS

The new COX-2 inhibitors have had dramatic results for some people. They provide the same pain relief as traditional NSAIDs but cause fewer ulcers. As a result, they may be of benefit if you cannot tolerate NSAIDs, have had an ulcer in the past, or are tired of taking antacids and other medications to prevent these problems from developing while taking NSAIDs. As many as one-third of the people with osteoarthritis who are taking prescription NSAIDs also need to take some other type of medication to counter the side effects.

Predictably, COX-2 inhibitors took off like a rocket in the marketplace. *Celebrex,* introduced in January 1999, soon became the most successful pharmaceutical launch to date, surpassing even the anti-impotence drug *Viagra.* But as time went on, some healthcare providers began to express caution about whether COX-2 inhibitors are appropriate for everyone.

RISKS OF COX-2 INHIBITORS

It is not yet known whether COX-2 inhibitors will reduce the serious complications of NSAIDs such as perforations or bleeding. Early results from clinical studies, however, appear positive.

COX-2 inhibitors are also not useful in preventing heart attacks and strokes, as is the case with traditional aspirin. Other questions will likely be raised and other risks identified for the new COX-2 inhibitors. In the meantime, though, the risk/benefit ratio seems to be tipped in favor of benefit. As always, it is best to consult with your healthcare provider before making any treatment decision. And you may want to consider cost as a factor: The COX-2 inhibitors can cost from $700 to $1,000 per year, depending on dose—and may be even more if you require a high dose (as for rheumatoid arthritis).

Corticosteroid Therapy

Corticosteroids are synthetic forms of naturally occurring hormones produced by the adrenal glands, which control your metabolism and your ability to absorb nutrients and excrete salt and water. Corticosteroids may be given as injections into the joints to treat flare-ups of rheumatoid arthritis or osteoarthritis. The injections provide short-term relief and reduce inflammation and pain while other medications become effective.

Low-dose corticosteroids in pill form are used for rheumatoid

arthritis, but generally not for osteoarthritis. Although corticosteroids can benefit patients, they also carry risks. For this reason
they should not be used for extended periods but for short-term
relief or as a "bridge" while waiting for other strategies to work.

More details on the use of corticosteroids to treat these types of
arthritis can be found in chapters 6 and 7.

Antidepressants

It may surprise you if your healthcare provider prescribes an
antidepressant when you are suffering from arthritis. Antidepressants may help you feel better. For one thing, they block nerve
pathways in the brain that are involved in both depression and pain.
Some antidepressants also prevent the breakdown of enkephalin,
believed to be one of the body's naturally produced pain-relieving
chemicals. Some may help you sleep better, which in turn makes
you better able to cope with pain.

Complementary Therapies

Perhaps you would like to supplement medical therapy with other
treatments that may not only alleviate pain but contribute to your
sense of well-being. These complementary, or alternative, therapies
may provide relief when used alone as well. Anecdotal evidence
indicates that these therapies are useful for many people, but clinical studies comparing one treatment to another have not been conducted to determine whether they are effective for the majority of
people. For more information about complementary therapies, see
chapter 11. You may also want to try some of the gentle movement
therapies explored in chapter 12.

For More Severe or Persistent Pain

If your pain does not respond to the medications just described, your healthcare provider may recommend several other options.

Nerve Blocks

If you have ever had Novocain at the dentist's office, you know what a nerve block is. This medication numbs a particular nerve to prevent a pain signal from getting through to your brain. Nerve blocks are effective at providing short-term relief and may even provide long-term relief in some patients. Be aware that in rare cases they can cause numbness and weakness around the injected area.

Transcutaneous Electrical Nerve Stimulation

A small device that sends electrical impulses to nerve endings just beneath the skin may relieve some pain. Transcutaneous electrical nerve stimulation (TENS) may work by preventing pain signals from getting through to your brain.

Narcotic Analgesics

These are more potent forms of analgesics and contain a narcotic, which may produce drowsiness. Although these do carry more risks than non-narcotic analgesics (most notably the chance of becoming addicted if you use them for a long time), they are prescribed when nothing else has worked.

Narcotic analgesics provide additional pain relief because they block certain chemical pathways that send pain signals through the central nervous system. But they also may create side effects in some people, including constipation, drowsiness, and nausea. The most frequently prescribed narcotic analgesics are acetaminophen with codeine (brand names include *Fioricet* and *Tylenol with Codeine*) and propoxyphene hydrochloride (*Darvon* and *Wygesic*).

In addition, a newer medication, tramadol *(Ultram)*, offers the benefits of narcotic analgesics but is not a narcotic.

Tranquilizers or Muscle Relaxants

Some patients think tranquilizers or muscle relaxants might relieve their pain. Muscle relaxants are used to relieve muscle tension and prevent painful spasms but generally when other strategies have failed. These medications may cause drowsiness or even depression, which can worsen your situation.

Talking to Your Healthcare Provider

No treatment decision is ever easy. This is especially true when deciding on the proper medication to take. There is no "right" answer most of the time; rather, the process involves a careful weighing of risks and benefits. The best approach is to start a conversation with your healthcare provider so that you can decide together what is the appropriate treatment for you.

Consult the Symptom Tracking Chart in chapter 4 for the type of information to give your healthcare provider. Also consider asking the following questions:

- What treatments do you recommend to alleviate my pain?
- What treatments will reduce my inflammation?
- What types of exercise is it safe for me to do?
- Can you recommend a self-help course? A support group?
- If a medication is prescribed, what is the brand name in the store? What is the generic name? Is the generic as effective as the brand name?
- How much should I take at one time and how often—in layman's terms (that is, not only in terms of milligrams per day but in number of tablets)?
- Is there a particular time of the day when I should take this medication?

- Should I take it with food or not? Any other suggestions on how best to take this medicine?
- How long will it be before I notice any benefits? How dramatic will the improvement be?
- How long will I have to take this medication? Weeks? Indefinitely?
- What are the most common side effects?
- What should I do if I notice them?
- What are the most dangerous side effects, the ones that should worry me?
- What do I do if I notice them? Whom can I contact and how? (Note: Physicians normally carry beepers so they can be reached when away from their offices, but check with your healthcare provider for advice about how to reach someone quickly.)
- How and where should I store the medicine so that it remains effective (that is, in refrigerator or cool cabinet)?
- What is the shelf life of the medicine (or the expiration date of the prescription)?
- How do I refill it? How many refills will the pharmacy provide before I need to come back for a visit?
- What does the medicine cost? How do I check to see if my health insurance plan covers it?

CHAPTER 6

Taking Charge of Osteoarthritis

The pain was so slight at first that Charles didn't notice it much. He'd feel an ache in his left knee when he got up in the morning, but it wasn't bad. He wasn't really sure when it started to get worse. It sort of crept up on him. One morning, as he stumbled getting off the bed, there was no denying it anymore: Something was wrong with that knee. It was so stiff that he had to limp to the bathroom.

By lunchtime his knee was moving fine, but the slight morning pain had become a throbbing ache. Charles grimaced as he sat down in the chair to call the doctor's office to schedule an appointment to have this looked at.

At sixty-eight you have to expect something would start going wrong, Charles figured. But why something that would interfere with his golf game?

IT IS said that there are only two certainties in life, death and taxes. Some would recommend adding a third if you live long enough: osteoarthritis.

Although statistics vary, X-ray examinations of joints show that most people who reach the age of seventy have osteoarthritis in at least one joint. Some experts even say that everyone over the age of sixty has osteoarthritis, although—for reasons that remain unclear—only some people develop symptoms such as pain.

Statistics also vary about the total number of people affected in the United States, but however you measure it, the population affected is sizable: anywhere from 16 million to 21 million. The disease is chronic, which means that once it develops, it will last for the rest of your life. And it has the potential to limit your activities severely. In fact, osteoarthritis is a leading source of disability in this country and by far the most common form of arthritis, accounting for almost as many cases as the other one hundred types of arthritis combined.

Yet in spite of being so common, osteoarthritis remains something of a medical puzzle. Although it is sometimes referred to as an inevitable part of aging, a function of prolonged wear and tear on your joints, it is not clear what causes the disease or how to prevent it.

But don't be overwhelmed or depressed if you have osteoarthritis. There is some good news, too, in the form of new clues about what causes it, identifiable risk factors (some of which can be modified), and effective treatments, with even more on the way. The past few years in particular have seen breakthroughs in the understanding and treatment of osteoarthritis. Certainly, if you have osteoarthritis, you can learn to manage the most bothersome symptoms and avoid disability. The key, as with many serious diseases, is early diagnosis and aggressive treatment. (For more information on diagnoses, see chapter 4.)

Osteoarthritis: More Than "Wear and Tear"

Anyone who has driven an old car over an unpaved road has some insight into the underlying problems in osteoarthritis. If the shock absorbers are worn out, the passengers in that old car will feel every bump and jolt. The ride might even become painful.

Cartilage is often called the body's shock absorber. This strong rubbery material covers the end of bones where they meet at joints. As bones move, the friction and grating that might otherwise occur when two hard materials collide are cushioned by the cartilage and a lubricating fluid from the surrounding synovial membrane. Osteoarthritis develops when the cartilage begins to wear out and loses its ability to cushion the bones. This leads to a gradual reshaping of the bone, which may eventually lead to deformity. As the disease progresses, the space between the bones within the joint area becomes smaller. At its most severe, bone might rub against bone.

Certainly the wear-and-tear analogy has its uses, and there is no question that repeated stress on the joint plays a role in the development of osteoarthritis. But this way of viewing osteoarthritis can also be misleading. Automobiles are built of mechanical parts that inevitably wear out after prolonged use. Your body, on the other hand, is a *biological* machine, built to constantly safeguard and repair its component parts.

Although we all change as we get older, osteoarthritis develops only when one of the underlying safety and maintenance systems goes awry. And the severity of the disease, which can range from mild to severe, probably depends on the interplay of a number of variables unrelated to age, such as gender, heredity, and physical activity. (See chapter 2 for more details about how cartilage is worn away and chapter 3 for more on risk factors.)

Thus, while the statistics just mentioned might give the impression that osteoarthritis is an inevitable part of aging, many researchers are not so sure. As the causes of this disease become clearer, so, too, do the chances that healthcare providers will find a way to intervene with the disease process before it develops or will be able to slow its progression. In the meantime, better understanding about the development of osteoarthritis has led to improved treatments, and more are on the way.

Symptoms

The initial symptoms of osteoarthritis may escape notice because they are so subtle and because they might happen in the course of an ordinary week, such as a little stiffness upon rising from bed in the morning or pain while performing routine daily tasks—opening a jar or pushing a vacuum. Sometimes the symptoms are dismissed as a sign of overwork or stress.

But what makes osteoarthritis symptoms different from a normal ache or pain are several things: duration (that is, it does not go away) and the way it interferes with daily activities on a regular basis. The types of joints usually affected are the hands, hips, knees, and spine. Generally, single joints are affected, but there is a sub-category of osteoarthritis in which the condition affects multiple joints or is *generalized*. Typical symptoms include the following:

PAIN

- Deep ache
- May not be specific to a particular part of your body
- Occurs in conjunction with activity if early in the day
- Occurs while resting if later in the day

STIFFNESS

- Have trouble moving affected joint but can move others
- Have trouble crouching
- Joint loosens up after fifteen to thirty minutes
- May worsen in certain types of weather

REDUCED RANGE OF MOTION

- Joint can no longer move to the extent it used to; it is harder to walk, reach for objects, or bend over

JOINT GIVES WAY

- Weight-bearing joints such as the hips and knees may give way when used

If these symptoms last more than several weeks, you may have osteoarthritis. Contact your healthcare provider to receive a diagnosis—the only way to know for sure.

Pain: The Most Common—and Vexing—Symptom

Pain in or around a joint is one of the most telltale symptoms of osteoarthritis. It is also one of the disease's most distressing aspects. (See chapter 5 for more details.)

Although it is the most commonly reported symptom, it does not affect everyone with the disease. Only about one-third of the people with evidence of mild osteoarthritis on an X ray will actually mention pain to their doctors, and it depends in part on the severity and location of the disease. In addition, people have varying pain thresholds, the point at which they will perceive pain, probably because of variations in their nervous systems.

At times the pain is a sentinel, sounding an alert and identifying the source of the problem. At other times it is a decoy, calling attention to one place when the real problem is somewhere else. Arthritis in the spinal cord may radiate upward to the neck and arms or downward to the legs. An arthritic hip may cause pain in the thigh, buttocks, groin, or even the knee. Such decoy pain is a *referred* pain because it occurs in a site other than the one injured or diseased. This happens because the various sensory nerves in different parts of the body come together as they wind their way toward the spinal cord, and so the brain may mistake the true source of pain.

The pain of osteoarthritis can be distinguished from other types of discomfort because it emanates from deep down rather than the surface. Maddeningly, the pain can come and go throughout the day and it can increase and decrease with different activities.

Other Symptoms

Bony protrusions. Some people with osteoarthritis develop bumps near the affected joint. They are sometimes visible beneath the surface of the skin, particularly on the hands. Sometimes the bumps themselves are not visible, but their presence beneath the surface of the skin makes an area seem swollen.

These bumps, or *osteophytes*, develop as the cartilage wears away and changes shape, and as greater pressure is placed on the bone and the marrow it contains. As a result, new bone is formed, typically on the sides of existing bone. Although not always visible to the naked eye, osteophytes can cause pain within the joint.

Swelling and inflammation. Swollen joints may be caused by synovial fluid that collects when the synovial membrane surrounding the joint has been irritated by bony protrusions or fragments of cartilage. The swelling may also be caused by inflammation, which causes the joint not only to swell, but also to become warm to the touch and to turn red. The joint may also be sore and tender when touched.

Inflammation results when your immune system responds to injury. Generally speaking, inflammation is not a major factor in osteoarthritis, but it sometimes occurs in this disease. Since inflammation is more directly involved in rheumatoid arthritis (see chapter 7), it is important to tell your healthcare provider if you experience this symptom.

How Symptoms May Vary Depending on Location

Although many of the same mechanisms are involved, osteoarthritis can cause different symptoms—and may even look different to an observer—depending on its location and whether it is generalized or confined to one joint.

HAND

Heberden's and *Bouchard's nodes* are types of osteoarthritis that develop in the hands. These nodes tend to occur in women over the age of fifty and appear as bony lumps at the end of the fingers. (See Heberden's and Bouchard's Nodes on page 114.) This type of arthritis tends to run in families, suggesting a genetic cause.

Another generalized form, erosive inflammatory osteoarthritis, erodes the finger joints. Inflammation results, which might be mistaken for a sign of rheumatoid arthritis. It can be distinguished from rheumatoid arthritis because other system wide symptoms are not present, such as fatigue, stiffness in all joints, and weight loss.

If you have osteoarthritis in your hand, you may have trouble opening jars or opening doors. It may hurt to turn the key in your car's ignition, and you may have trouble completing the motion. You may start having trouble buttoning your shirts or zipping up a skirt. If you begin to notice such symptoms, talk with your healthcare provider.

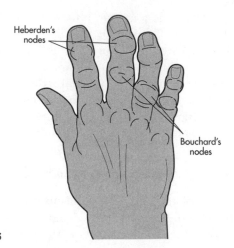

Heberden's
nodes

Bouchard's
nodes

Heberden's and Bouchard's Nodes

HIP

The hips are surrounded by nerves—the femoral, sciatic, and obturator. This means that pain caused by an osteoarthritic hip may not always be felt in the hip joint itself but may be felt nearby. An arthritic hip most often causes pain in the groin, but you may also feel pain in your buttocks, thigh, or knee.

The pain caused by an arthritic hip builds slowly with time, usually over several months or even years, and you may feel it as a dull ache. As the arthritis progresses in the hip, it may affect your ability to walk; typically, people try to favor the affected leg, taking only a short stride. You may also have difficulty putting on your shoes or socks. Walking up stairs may be more painful than walking on level ground. You may have trouble getting up from the toilet seat or a chair. If you begin to notice these symptoms, contact your health-care provider.

KNEE

If you have osteoarthritis of the knee, you are likely to feel the pain in your knee, although on occasion it will be felt in the hip area. When at rest, your knee might feel stiff. Once you start to move, your knee might hurt but eventually loosen up. Pain may increase when you climb or descend stairs, or after prolonged periods of standing or walking. Swelling is more likely to be present in your knee than in other joints.

SPINE

Back pain is common, affecting as many as 80 percent of American adults at one time or another. Pain that is the result of osteoarthritis produces a deep and persistent ache at any point along the spine and may produce stiffness as cartilage wears away and flexibility is lost. Occasionally the pain radiates to your neck or buttocks as nerves become compressed. A backache that persists beyond a few days may be a sign of osteoarthritis. Contact your healthcare provider.

Diagnosing Osteoarthritis

Diagnosis is particularly important in osteoarthritis because there are so many individual variations of the disease. That means the best treatment plan for your particular situation may be quite different from someone else's.

It is also important to note that while most people with osteoarthritis will feel pain, not everyone experiencing pain has osteoarthritis. In particular, pain that is bad enough to awaken you from sleep could be a sign of soft tissue inflammation, as with bursitis and tendinitis, or of significant joint damage, a bone fracture, or even nerve entrapment. If you are awakened by pain, mention this to your healthcare provider.

To determine whether your symptoms are signs of osteoarthritis or something else, your healthcare provider will look at the following:

- Your medical history—the information you provide about duration and type of symptoms
- The results of a physical examination
- The results of X rays and other medical tests

General information about these diagnostic techniques is contained in chapter 4. When osteoarthritis is suspected, your healthcare provider may conduct the following tests:

X ray. Your healthcare provider may ask a radiologist to take an X ray of the affected joint to provide a clearer picture of what is going on beneath the skin.

An X ray may be needed if your healthcare provider wants to confirm the diagnosis or if it is in question. X rays may also be required for the hips and knees, especially if your healthcare provider wants to provide diagnostic information about the degree of joint space narrowing that cannot otherwise be determined. And X rays are always needed if your healthcare provider is contemplating recommending orthopedic surgery.

If your healthcare provider is confident about your diagnosis, an X ray may not be needed. In osteoarthritis the X ray is almost always abnormal by the time you feel symptoms such as pain, so there may be no need to take one. And X rays are generally not needed to diagnose osteoarthritis of the hands because visual inspection and palpation can usually confirm a diagnosis.

Blood sample. Your healthcare provider may also want to take a blood sample, to determine if you are a candidate for treatment with NSAIDs (which are discussed in greater detail in chapter 5). He or she may request a complete blood count and liver and kidney function tests to ensure that NSAIDs are appropriate for you. If your healthcare provider believes you are suffering from other types of arthritis, other blood tests may be done. If there is swelling in the joint or if the diagnosis is in question, your healthcare provider may also withdraw fluid from the joint for diagnostic purposes.

Managing the Symptoms

Although there is no way to cure osteoarthritis, you can certainly learn to manage the disease and prevent it from disabling you. A multifaceted treatment plan can help reduce pain, maintain or improve your mobility, and improve your overall health.

Once your healthcare provider has diagnosed osteoarthritis, he or she will work with you to develop a treatment plan so that you can manage your symptoms. The specific treatment plan you choose will depend on the level of pain you are experiencing, how much your arthritis is interfering with your day-to-day life, and sometimes on the extent of joint damage as revealed in an X ray.

For milder forms of osteoarthritis you may be able to manage your symptoms by paying better attention to diet and exercise (see chapter 3 for more details). Treatment for more advanced disease will consist of some type of medication or pharmacologic agent as well as other elements such as diet, physical therapy, complementary therapy, and, for the most severe cases, even surgery.

Fundamentals of a Treatment Plan

Learn about osteoarthritis. Education is often the first step in learning to manage your osteoarthritis. As mentioned in chapter 4, education is what will empower you as a patient. The more you know about osteoarthritis, the better you will understand the symptoms and treatment options. Even better, studies have shown that people who educate themselves about arthritis and learn to manage their symptoms say they have less joint pain and visit their healthcare providers less often, while their level of physical activity and overall quality of life are improved. You could be one of them!

Your healthcare provider should have brochures and pamphlets about the disease to share with you. If not, ask how you can obtain them. Videos and pamphlets about osteoarthritis are available, often free of charge, from organizations such as The Arthritis Foundation.

Find support. The Arthritis Foundation has local chapters all over the country, and many of its members suffer from osteoarthritis. They can provide the moral support you will need occasionally, especially if your disease is advanced. Or you might ask your healthcare provider if your hospital or clinic offers a support group for people with osteoarthritis.

Lose weight. A number of studies have shown that if you lose weight, you will feel less pain from your osteoarthritis and will be able to move more easily. The reason? Less weight means less pressure on your joints, and they're already facing enough pressure as it is. Just walking down the street places a force equal to roughly three times your weight on the joints in the lower portion of your body (see chapter 2). So by losing even 5 pounds you can eliminate 15 pounds of pressure on your knees and ankles with each step.

Although a new diet fad seems to hit the country once a month, there is a deceptively simple formula for losing weight: Burn more calories than you eat every day. That doesn't mean you should starve. In fact, when you have osteoarthritis, it's time to pay more attention to nutrition so that you have the energy you'll need to cope with symptoms.

The fundamentals of a good diet are contained in chapter 3. When you have osteoarthritis, the following points are especially important:

- Eat less fat and sugar. This is the time to start substituting a bagel for a muffin at breakfast, for instance. Or substitute fish for meat several times a week. Read the labels on "low-fat" pastries carefully. Many are so loaded with sugar that you end up gaining weight without expecting to.
- Eat more vegetables and fruits. You should try to eat at least five servings of fruits and vegetables a day. Not only will this provide you with the vitamins and nutrients you need, but it will also help you avoid cookies, potato chips, and other high-fat choices.
- Eat plenty of whole-grain products. Whole-grain breads, dried beans, and certain types of cereal provide fiber, which helps you digest food better.

For more information on how to adapt your diet once you have arthritis, see chapter 12.

Exercise. If done regularly and in a way that protects your joints, exercise will reduce your pain and improve your mobility. The challenge once you have osteoarthritis is to start slow and pay special attention to your affected joints.

As explained previously, an overall fitness plan consists of range-of-motion exercises to improve flexibility, resistance exercises to strengthen muscles, and aerobic exercises to build heart and lung function and endurance. The type of exercises you do will depend on the joints affected by osteoarthritis.

If you have osteoarthritis of the knee or anywhere else below the waist, avoid high-impact exercises such as running, tennis, and basketball. This may be the time to switch to leisurely bicycling and walking, which don't jolt the joints in the lower part of your body as much as other exercises.

Probably the best type of exercise is swimming because the water supports your weight and removes any harsh impact on your joints. If you have osteoarthritis in your hands or shoulders, you can do gentle range-of-motion exercises, but it may be time to stop lifting weights. No matter what type of exercises you choose, start with gentle range-of-motion exercises to increase your flexibility.

To help alleviate pain, it's helpful to strengthen the muscles surrounding your affected joint. If your joint is really hurting, then isometric exercises may help. In *isometric* exercises you tighten and then relax specific muscle groups without actually moving your joint. In *isotonic* exercises, you strengthen your muscles by moving a particular joint repeatedly.

If you have osteoarthritis in your knee, for instance, you may benefit from strengthening the quadriceps in your leg (located at the front of your thigh, it supports your knee). If your knee is sore, try the isometric exercise on page 120. If you are able to move your knee without too much pain, try the isotonic exercise on page 121. Both exercises will build your quadriceps muscle.

If you have osteoarthritis of the hip, you may find that walking or climbing the stairs is difficult. To improve your hip motion and the strength of the supporting muscles, try these exercises from The

Isometric Exercise

To strengthen your leg muscles while protecting your knee joints, try this exercise. While seated, cross your ankles in front of you. Squeeze your shins together, thrusting forward with your back leg while pulling backward with your front leg. Keep squeezing your legs together, without moving your feet, for 10 seconds, then relax. Switch legs and repeat.

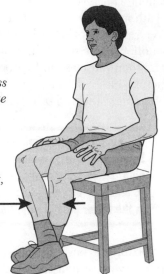

Arthritis Foundation. Repeat each exercise three to twelve times. (For additional suggestions, see chapter 12.)

KNEE LIFTS

1. Sit in a chair, making sure that your back is straight.
2. Lift your right knee and slowly bring it up toward your chest. You can grasp the front of your knee or clasp your thigh underneath to help.
3. Hold for a few seconds, then release.
4. Repeat with the left knee.

LEG/HIP ROTATIONS

1. Hold the back of a chair for support (a chair that is about waist level is perfect).
2. While keeping your knee straight, swing your right leg to the front, side, and back.
3. Repeat. (You can bend your other knee if it helps.)

Isometric Exercise

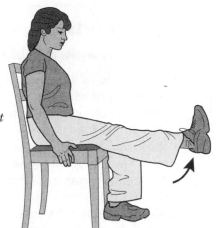

One way to strengthen the quadriceps muscles, which help support your knee, is to do this exercise. While seated, raise your right leg slowly until it is straight out in front of you. Hold the position for 5 seconds, then slowly relax the position and let your foot return to the ground. Now do the same with your left leg.

4. With your right leg resting lightly on the floor, place your weight on your left leg.
5. Move your right leg from your hip so that your right knee and foot point first inward then outward (as if you were rubbing something out).
6. Repeat the exercise for your left leg.

Support your joints. To take the pressure off your affected joints or to provide them with extra support, look into assistive or adaptive devices. Using a cane temporarily can help reduce the strain on your knee, for instance. Wedged insoles for your shoes will help absorb the impact of each step and may also adjust for any misalignment that has occurred as a result of your injured joints. Splints and braces help keep joints in proper alignment and distribute weight more evenly.

You can find many of these devices at your local pharmacy, but it's best to consult with your healthcare provider first. Using the wrong device or wearing one that is not fitted properly may hurt you more than help you. For more information see chapter 10.

Seek physical therapy. Physical therapy and its close cousin, occupational therapy, will help you regain some of the mobility

Tips for Exercising with Osteoarthritis

To make it easier on your joints, try the following approaches:

- Take a warm bath or shower before you exercise. This helps your muscles relax and reduces pain.
- If one of your joints is particularly sore, apply a cold pack or a heating pad to the area. Both methods will help reduce pain.
- Start slowly. Although ideally you should get 30 minutes of aerobic exercise a day, that may seem overwhelming at first. You can get just as much benefit from several 10-minute workouts a day.
- When working on strength exercises to build muscles, go easy on your joints. If you are working with weights, decrease the weight you're using but increase the number of repetitions to build your muscle.
- Be sure to protect your back so that you don't strain it. Many exercises can be performed while sitting or holding on to a chair.

Stop exercising immediately if

- You suffer chest pain
- You become dizzy or short of breath
- You become nauseous
- Your pain becomes worse while doing an exercise

For additional suggestions, see chapter 12.

you have lost and teach you to protect yourself against further joint damage. It is best to consult a physical therapist as soon as you are diagnosed because early intervention may produce a better outcome.

One of the first things that happens when you develop osteoarthritis is that it becomes more difficult to move the affected joint. But if you don't move it, your muscles will weaken and only complicate the problem. So start with some gentle range-of-motion exercises to maintain flexibility and then try some isometric exercises to build up the muscle without straining your joints.

As you feel more confident using the joint, add aerobic activities to your routine. This can be as simple as taking a walk or riding a bicycle. Another excellent exercise is swimming, which will get your heart and lungs working without straining your joints.

More information about physical and occupational therapy, and exercises you can do at home, will be discussed in chapter 10.

Medication Strategies

If the pain persists, if your osteoarthritis has already progressed to a more advanced stage, or if it involves more than one joint, then your healthcare provider will likely recommend some type of medication.

Most types of medications discussed here are *systemic* in effect, meaning that they circulate in the bloodstream and therefore may affect areas other than the joints. Side effects vary from person to person; for this reason it is important to let your healthcare provider know whether you are experiencing any side effects and whether you think the medication is helping to reduce your symptoms.

It is important to remember that any medication requires time to become effective, ranging from several hours to several months depending on the agent.

And check your health insurance coverage to find out how much you have to pay for a particular medication. This is rapidly becoming one of the most contentious and complicated parts of therapy. For a comparative look at costs, see Table 7. For tips on health insurance coverage, see Table 3 on page 90.

TABLE 7. **Comparing Costs**

Type of Medication	Estimated Cost
Analgesics (*Anacin, Darvon, Tylenol*)	Range from $120/year for OTC medications to $1,400/year for prescription medications
NSAIDs (*Arthrotec, Daypro,* ibuprofen)	Range from $100/year for OTC medications to $500 to $1,100/year for prescription medications
COX-2 inhibitors (*Celebrex, Vioxx*)	$700–$1,000/year (Costs may be higher if you require a large dose.)
Corticosteroid injections	$20 to $30 for the corticosteroids plus physician charges to inject
Hyaluronic acid injections (*Hyalgan, Synvisc*)	$500–$635 per series plus physician charges to inject

Note: All costs are estimates based on average use.

For Mild to Moderate Pain

If you have mild to moderate pain from arthritis, work with your healthcare provider to find the best medication strategy. The approach you choose will depend on a number of factors, including the amount of pain you are feeling, how much it is interfering with your day-to-day activities, your view of medications in general, and your budget and health insurance coverage. As mentioned in chapter 5, there is no "one size fits all" when it comes to any part of a treatment plan. This is especially true of decisions regarding medication.

The first suggestion by your healthcare provider may be an over-the-counter medication. In the treatment of osteoarthritis, as in the treatment of any disease, healthcare providers prefer to start with the simplest medicines that carry the least amount of side effects and then increase the aggressiveness of treatment as the situation warrants.

ANALGESICS

If you have mild to moderate pain in your joints, similar to that from a headache or toothache, you might want to consider taking analgesics, medications that relieve pain without reducing inflammation. Acetaminophen, one of the most commonly used analgesics, is the active ingredient in a number of over-the-counter medications, including brand names such as aspirin-free *Anacin*, *Excedrin*, and *Tylenol*.

Generally a dose of 3,000 to 4,000 milligrams a day (equivalent to six to eight 500-milligram tablets of *Tylenol*) is required to relieve the pain of osteoarthritis. This should be safe unless you have liver disease or drink alcohol excessively.

For some people with osteoarthritis, acetaminophen may be the only treatment needed; for others, this medication may be combined with an anti-inflammatory agent. For more information about analgesics, see chapter 5.

TOPICAL ANALGESICS

Topical analgesics (available in creams, lotions, or gels) provide pain relief to a particular joint or joints after being applied to the surface of the skin. If you have mild osteoarthritis pain that is limited to one or two joints, or if you want to supplement the effectiveness of an oral medication, then you may want to try topical analgesics.

NON-STEROIDAL ANTI-INFLAMMATORY DRUGS (NSAIDs)

If you do not experience adequate pain relief from acetaminophen, you may want to talk with your healthcare provider about NSAIDs. At low doses NSAIDs relieve pain, at higher doses they also reduce inflammation. Since inflammation is not generally a problem in osteoarthritis, the NSAIDs may be prescribed at lower doses, and their side effects may not be troublesome. But if your pain is severe or if you also have inflammation, your healthcare provider might prescribe higher doses of any given NSAIDs.

The NSAID family of medications includes aspirin, ibuoprofen (brand names include *Advil* and *Motrin*), and naproxen. Because this family of medications does carry some risk of gastrointestinal upset and bleeding, talk about the relative risks and benefits with your healthcare provider. He or she may order some blood tests to determine whether or not NSAIDs are appropriate for you or may recommend that you combine the NSAID with another medication that will protect your stomach. More information on this class of medication is provided in chapter 5.

COX-2 INHIBITORS

If you are at high risk for suffering gastrointestinal upset or stomach bleeding, or if you have had an ulcer, talk with your healthcare provider about one of the new COX-2 inhibitors. These new medications are types of NSAIDs that can alleviate pain with fewer stomach side effects than aspirin or other NSAIDs.

COX-2 inhibitors act only on the COX-2 enzyme, which causes pain and inflammation, while ignoring COX-1, which is involved in protecting the lining of the stomach. In doing so, the COX-2 inhibitors appear to reduce a common side effect of NSAIDs: gastrointestinal ulcers.

Celecoxib, marketed under the brand name *Celebrex,* and rofecoxib, marketed as *Vioxx,* have been approved by the FDA. Others are in various stages of development. See chapter 5 for more information.

INJECTIONS OF CORTICOSTEROIDS

If you have mild to moderate arthritis pain and have not responded well to treatment with acetaminophen, your doctor may recommend injections of corticosteroids, which provide short-term relief and reduce inflammation and pain while other medications become effective.

Steroid use may conjure up images of muscle-heavy athletes artificially bulking up on hormones to achieve super-human strength. But the steroids that some athletes use are derived from the male sex hormone, testosterone, whereas corticosteroids are synthetic versions of hormones produced by the adrenal glands. An entirely different type of steroid, they have proven useful in the treatment of osteoarthritis of the knee as well as in rheumatoid arthritis. Corticosteroids have been used for intra-articular injection, or within the joint, since the 1950s. Since then, their popularity as a treatment for osteoarthritis has ebbed and flowed.

Taking corticosteroids in pill form is not recommended for you if you have osteoarthritis.

The injections are done in your healthcare provider's office. He or she will first remove excess fluid from your joint and then inject the corticosteroids directly into the area.

Although such injections can alleviate pain, too many injections may actually damage your joints. For this reason it is recommended that such injections be given only three or four times a year.

HYALURONIC ACID

If you have osteoarthritis of the knee and other strategies have not provided relief, your healthcare provider may suggest hyaluronic acid injections.

Hyaluronic acid is a naturally occurring substance in cartilage and the synovial fluid that surrounds it. If you have osteoarthritis, both your cartilage and joint fluid degrade over time.

Since the 1970s a type of hyaluronic acid has been injected into racehorses with osteoarthritis. The FDA recently approved a similar treatment for people. Two medications, hyaluronan (brand name *Hyalgan*) and hylan G-F20 (brand name *Synvisc*) have been approved by the FDA for osteoarthritis of the knee.

Both medications serve as a substitute for the naturally occurring hyaluronan, which is a component in your joint fluid that contributes to its thick, syrupy qualities.

Although hyaluronic acid injections do appear to help lubricate the joint area temporarily, the major benefit of such an injection is pain relief: It may alleviate pain for up to one year. There is also some evidence that these injections may improve mobility. There is no proof, though, that hyaluronic acid injections will slow the progression of the disease or repair the damage already done.

Generally, hyaluronic acid injections are given once a week for a period of three to five weeks, depending on the medication chosen. These injections are usually given by rheumatologists or orthopedic surgeons who have advanced training in joint disease and its treatment. The area is usually numbed ahead of time with a local anesthetic. If your knee is swollen, your joint fluid may be removed before hyaluronic acid is injected.

It is not known exactly how hyaluronic acid injections work. The cumulative therapeutic effect seems to result from a combination of anti-inflammatory action, better lubrication (at least for a short period), pain relief by directly acting on synovial nerve endings, and stimulating the synovial lining in a way that produces naturally occurring hyaluronic acid.

This treatment is not recommended for anyone with an infection, rash, or other type of skin disorder at the site of the injection. If you are allergic to egg products, you should mention this to your healthcare provider.

TETRACYCLINES

Long valued for their effect on fighting infections, the family of medications known as tetracyclines is receiving renewed appreciation for their potential to treat osteoarthritis. Although best known for their ability to neutralize invading microbes, these medications also appear to inhibit two key players in the destruction of cartilage: metalloproteinases and collagenase.

Doxycycline and minocycline, types of tetracycline that have been used to treat acne, are currently being studied for osteoarthritis. In animal studies, doxycycline slowed the degradation of cartilage and reduced the damage done by osteoarthritis. Other studies have shown that doxycycline helps maintain the cartilage's own built-in repair mechanisms and thus extend its health.

For More Severe Pain

If your pain is severe and does not respond to other therapies, your healthcare provider may recommend more potent therapies, including narcotic medications. Although none were specifically developed to treat osteoarthritis, and they do carry more risks than non-narcotic analgesics, many healthcare providers will prescribe them if nothing else has worked.

Narcotic analgesics provide additional relief because they work through the central nervous system to prevent pain signals both from being sent and received. The most frequently prescribed narcotic analgesics are acetaminophen with codeine (*Fioricet* and *Tylenol with Codeine*) and propoxyphene hydrochloride (*Darvon* and *Wygesic*).

The disadvantage of any medication containing a narcotic is that it can become addictive. For this reason it is best to monitor your doses carefully and work with your healthcare provider to avoid becoming addicted.

In addition, a newer medication, tramadol, offers the benefits of narcotic analgesics even though it does not appear to be addictive. Tramadol may be appropriate for you if you have moderate to severe pain from osteoarthritis, have not responded to other therapies, or are not able to take NSAIDs or COX-2 inhibitors for some reason.

If you require narcotic medications to treat your pain, you should make an appointment to see a rheumatologist. He or she may be able to adjust your medication to improve the amount of pain relief you experience. A rheumatologist will also be able to evaluate your joint and determine whether surgery might be appropriate.

Therapies Under Investigation

New therapies for osteoarthritis are being investigated all the time. Because it can take years to conduct the rigorous clinical trials that determine whether a new treatment is effective or not, it is possible you may hear about a new therapy and wonder if it is appropriate for you.

For example, gene therapy is a broad and rapidly evolving field of medicine that offers a whole new approach to treating diseases like arthritis. In this approach a therapeutic agent is introduced into the cells of a joint in the hope that the body will begin reproducing the agent and actually begin to fix the damage caused by arthritis. A number of investigations are now under way to determine if gene therapy would be helpful in treating osteoarthritis. Researchers are investigating whether this technique can be used to help repair cartilage damaged by osteoarthritis or prevent the damage from occurring in the first place by blocking certain cells in the synovial fluid. But don't expect any new treatment soon. Gene therapy faces a number of challenges, including finding ways to transfer genes to the target site and then to activate them once they are there. Still, this is definitely a field to watch.

Another therapy is tidal irrigation of the joint, which involves the withdrawal of joint fluid followed by lavage (a type of wash) with a saline solution. It is being investigated for people who have osteoarthritis of the knee and have not responded to other treatments. Clinical trials are currently under way.

Complementary Therapies

Some people find it helpful to add one or more complementary therapies to whatever strategy they are using to manage their osteoarthritis. Therapies such as acupuncture may alleviate pain, while others such as tai chi may help restore movement as well as reduce pain.

Glucosamine and chondroitin sulfate supplements have generated a lot of interest among people with osteoarthritis. (Generally people take 1,500 milligrams of glucosamine or 1,200 milligrams of chondroitin sulfate a day.) Early studies have reported that these supplements ease the pain of osteoarthritis. They have been used in Europe for years. Large clinical studies are being performed in the United States and Europe to determine their effect on disease progression. See chapter 11 for more information.

Whatever complementary approaches you decide to use, make sure you mention them to your healthcare provider. As safe as many of these remedies may seem, it's always best to see if there are any therapies you should avoid. For instance, yoga may be wonderful, but if you have osteoarthritis, you may have to skip certain postures. And if you have a shellfish allergy, you may not want to take certain supplements, such as glucosamine, that are derived from crab and lobster shells.

Herbs, vitamins, and other dietary supplements are not regulated by the FDA, so the quality of these products may vary. Just because the packaging lists a particular set of ingredients does not guarantee that all of them are included in the quantities listed. And the highly popular glucosamine and chondroitin sulfate supplements use different types of active ingredients. Some chondroitin sulfate supplements are derived from cattle trachea (perfectly acceptable); others are made from shark cartilage (not recommended because they may be contaminated with heavy metals).

Surgery

If you have severe pain and other symptoms of osteoarthritis, and nothing else has worked, make an appointment to see a rheumatologist. He or she can determine if it is worth your while to see an orthopedic surgeon. Since your rheumatologist is not a surgeon, this visit can also serve as a second opinion about whether you need surgery.

There are several surgical options you can consider. Arthroscopy, a minimally invasive surgery, can be helpful for your knee or shoulders. An osteotomy can be performed to realign bones. Total joint replacement, especially for your knee or hip, can eliminate pain and restore function. For more information see chapter 13.

CHAPTER 7

Taking Charge of Rheumatoid Arthritis

Turning forty wasn't supposed to be this bad.

For the past few months Marjorie felt stiff and sore when she got out of bed in the morning—the way she used to feel after helping someone move or after cleaning out the basement. It could take a good hour or so for her to limber up, but by lunchtime she'd feel worn out and ready for a nap. This was not the kind of thing her boss understood.

She also noticed that her wrists and knuckles became swollen and sore, making it hard to move her hands. Initially, the pain went away after taking a couple of aspirin, but lately that didn't seem to help. Marjorie did a lot of word processing work at her job and wondered if this could be the beginning of carpal tunnel syndrome.

But the last straw was when both of her knees felt sore and started to swell and turn red. Now even tennis, the sport that helped her unwind at the end of a long day, had become something she thought twice about. What was going on? What could this be?

Marjorie was even more surprised when her healthcare provider decided it might be rheumatoid arthritis and suggested she see a rheumatologist.

ALTHOUGH RHEUMATOID arthritis has traditionally been one of the most disabling types of arthritis, it may surprise you to learn how much optimism currently exists about the prospects for people who develop this disease. The past few years in particular have seen several significant developments, both in understanding this disease and in treating it. In fact, rheumatoid arthritis has become one of the most exciting areas in arthritis care and research.

While no one is talking cure yet, these developments have certainly provided more choices for you if you have rheumatoid arthritis—especially if you are newly diagnosed. The key is to begin treatment with a specialist as early as possible.

Why a specialist? Rheumatoid arthritis is a complex and rapidly advancing disease. To ensure that you fare as well as possible, consult with someone who has advanced training and has kept up with current developments. A rheumatologist is a specialist in the care of bone and joint diseases who will be aware of the latest research in the field and will have a great deal of experience treating people with conditions similar to yours. (See chapter 4 for more information about rheumatologists.)

So whether you notice the telltale symptoms first or your primary care provider makes the preliminary diagnosis, it is best to consult with a rheumatologist. And the earlier you see a rheumatologist, the better. Although we used to take a wait-and-see approach to treating rheumatoid arthritis—forestalling aggressive therapies until X rays provided evidence of joint destruction—earlier intervention is now recommended.

Recent studies have shown that joint damage begins much earlier than previously suspected, and certainly before it is evident on an X ray. So early, aggressive treatment—ideally within one year after onset of the disease—is the best way to prevent the disability that rheumatoid arthritis can cause.

As always, though, the final treatment strategy you choose will depend on your particular form of the disease, health profile, and preferences. This chapter is intended to help you better understand rheumatoid arthritis, provide some tips on how to help yourself, and explain the treatment options available so that you can better discuss them with your rheumatologist.

What Is Rheumatoid Arthritis?

Rheumatoid arthritis develops when your own immune system attacks parts of your body. It is not clear why the immune system goes awry in rheumatoid arthritis. Chief suspects include a genetic profile that might make you susceptible to the disease and exposure to infectious agents that initiate an immune attack. See chapter 2 for more details.

The disease affects more than 2 million people in the United States, about 1 percent of the population. Rheumatoid arthritis can affect anyone—men and women, young and old, regardless of race or where you live. But it usually develops in people between the ages of twenty and fifty. Women are two to three times as likely to develop the disease as men, for reasons that remain unclear.

Because the disease is systemic, it may eventually affect other parts of the body besides the joints and can adversely affect your health. Fortunately, new treatments provide options that didn't exist a few years ago.

Joints Affected

One of the distinguishing features of rheumatoid arthritis is the number and types of joints affected. Unlike osteoarthritis, which typically affects one joint at a time, rheumatoid arthritis tends to affect several joints at once. And generally the same joint on both sides of the body will be affected at the same time. For instance, if one elbow is affected, it is likely the other elbow will be as well.

The disease affects only the mobile joints, the ones such as the knee and wrist that enable you to move. (Fixed joints, such as those that connect the bones in the skull, do not move.) Mobile joints are surrounded by a synovial membrane, a protective covering that produces a slippery substance known as synovial fluid that lubricates the joint and facilitates movement.

Most often, rheumatoid arthritis affects the ankles, elbows, feet, hands, hips, jaw, knees, neck, and shoulders. It tends not to affect the lower spine.

Symptoms

Symptoms of rheumatoid arthritis differ from one person to the next. Even so, there are certain hallmark signs of the disease.

The more obvious symptoms—swollen or deformed joints, reduced movement and pain—occur as the disease progresses. Early symptoms can be much more subtle. Nevertheless, recent research has shown that, even as early as a year or two after onset of the disease, rheumatoid arthritis can cause irreversible destruction of joints. For that reason rheumatologists urge primary care providers and others to stay alert to the early signs of rheumatoid arthritis. The earlier that treatment begins, the better the chance of avoiding disability.

The subtle early symptoms that might easily be mistaken for something else include:

- Listlessness and fatigue
- Loss of appetite
- Soreness and some swelling in the joints
- Weight loss
- Joint stiffness, especially in the morning

As the Disease Progresses

Rheumatoid arthritis almost always eventually causes joints to become inflamed, making them sore and warm to the touch. The area may swell and turn red. The joints may become painful and hard to move.

Although joint inflammation is a hallmark sign of rheumatoid arthritis, it can vary from one person to another. In some people, joint inflammation flares up and then subsides, only to flare up again. In others, inflammation is always present and may even worsen as the disease progresses. About one person in ten experiences a single episode of joint inflammation and then goes into remission.

As the disease progresses, rheumatoid arthritis may also create flu-like symptoms. You may feel listless and weak, run a low-grade fever, and have no appetite. In time this may lead to weight loss and anemia.

Less often, symptoms of rheumatoid arthritis include inflamed tendons and tingling in the fingers. In about one person out of five, small bumps, known as nodules, appear under the skin on the elbows or on other parts of the body. These nodules are actually small lumps of tissue which develop around bony areas that are exposed to pressure. Though rare, these bumps may develop anywhere on the body and even internally.

Impact on Day-to-Day Activities

You may begin to have trouble getting dressed in the morning; your hands fumble at your buttons or you drop a hanger while trying to pull it out of the closet. It may be harder to get in and out of the shower or to reach around to wash your back. At work you may be able to use the keyboard of your computer without difficulty but be unable to hold your pen.

It is important to note these changes as well as the physical ones mentioned earlier. Not only will this help your rheumatologist determine how advanced your rheumatoid arthritis is, but it will also pinpoint activities that you may need to rethink and even learn how to do differently so that you can continue to live a full life.

It is possible to recover function. Just as the physical symptoms of your disease will require medication, the life-altering aspects can be addressed in other ways. But first you have to note them.

Signs of Advanced or Severe Disease

If you have a particularly severe form of rheumatoid arthritis or if the disease has progressed unchecked, your joints may become deformed. In some cases the disease may also involve other areas:

- Tissue in the eyes and mouth may become dry (Sjögren's syndrome)

- The tissues surrounding the heart may become inflamed (pericarditis)
- The tissues lining the lungs may become inflamed (pleuritis)

Rarely, rheumatoid arthritis affects blood vessels in a condition known as vasculitis. If this happens, the skin, nerves, organs, and other tissues may be damaged.

Diagnosis of Rheumatoid Arthritis

Diagnosis is all the more challenging because rheumatoid arthritis causes different symptoms in different people. To further complicate the situation, some symptoms—particularly pain and stiffness in the joints—are also symptoms of osteoarthritis. The feeling of overall weakness and lack of energy are symptoms of other autoimmune disorders such as lupus. To ensure that a diagnosis of rheumatoid arthritis is accurate, your rheumatologist will order various medical tests to supplement what he or she observes and what you have said about your symptoms.

To determine whether the symptoms are signs of rheumatoid arthritis or something else, your rheumatologist will look at the following:

- Your medical history—the information you provide about duration and type of symptoms
- The results of a physical examination
- The results of blood tests, X rays, and other medical tests

Medical History and Physical Examination

Your rheumatologist will ask you about your medical history and do a physical examination. See chapter 4, which covers these components of a diagnosis and has the Symptom Tracking Chart which you may want to start using to better prepare for your visit.

Don't be alarmed if your healthcare provider suggests that you return periodically for in-depth checkups that may involve many of the same questions and tests. Because rheumatoid arthritis can vary so much from one person to the next, time and reassessment offer valuable perspectives about the course of the disease.

Medical Tests

Although medical tests are also covered in chapter 4, the types of tests ordered when rheumatoid arthritis is suspected may vary from the tests ordered for the diagnosis of other types of arthritis.

BLOOD TESTS

A blood test is ordered in most cases. Unfortunately, no blood test can confirm or rule out a diagnosis of rheumatoid arthritis, but the tests are valuable in providing evidence that will point to the disease, or away from it.

Rheumatoid factor testing. Antibodies are synthesized when the body is fighting an infection; they are produced by specialized immune system cells known as lymphocytes and travel through the bloodstream to the site of an infection. One such antibody is called the rheumatoid factor and blood tests will reveal whether you have it.

In rheumatoid arthritis, however, antibodies may form even when there is no infection. The rheumatoid factor is found in the blood of about 80 percent of people with rheumatoid arthritis; however, 10 percent of people *without* rheumatoid arthritis test positive for rheumatoid factor. At the same time, you can have rheumatoid arthritis and not have a rheumatoid factor, so the presence or absence of this factor is not enough to make a diagnosis one way or another.

Erythrocyte sedimentation rate ("sed rate," or ESR). This blood test (not just used for rheumatoid arthritis) provides an indirect measure of inflammation and can be used to determine the activity rate of your rheumatoid arthritis. The higher the sedimentation rate, the more likely inflammation, a sign of rheumatoid arthritis, is present.

Plasma viscosity, or C-reactive protein (CRP). This blood test may be used instead of the sedimentation rate test because it is a more sensitive measure of inflammation.

Other Tests

Joint aspiration or arthrocentesis. In this procedure your rheumatologist will remove, or aspirate, a small amount of synovial fluid from your joint. The fluid can then be analyzed in a laboratory to rule out other diseases.

X rays. A radiologist may take an X ray of the affected joint or joints to give the rheumatologist a clearer picture of what is going on beneath the skin. In rheumatoid arthritis, X rays not only help with diagnosis, but may also be requested periodically to determine the progress of the disease. X rays are always needed if orthopedic surgery is being considered.

Health Status Measurements

Your rheumatologist may also ask you to fill out some type of health status measurement to determine the impact of your rheumatoid arthritis on your day-to-day activities. This will help to determine how advanced your rheumatoid arthritis is and how it is affecting the functioning of your joints. It will also be helpful in suggesting exercise and physical or occupational therapy. Once you start a treatment plan, it will also enable you to "measure" progress in a way that may mean more to you than the results of your blood test. For a sample health status measurement, see Table 8.

TABLE 8. **Health Assessment Questionnaire**

Date performed: _____

Key
0 = Without any difficulty
1 = With some difficulty
2 = With help from another person
3 = Unable to do

Are you able to:
I.   **Dressing and grooming**
    a. Get your clothes out of the closet and drawers?   _____
    b. Dress yourself, including tying your shoelaces and doing buttons? _____
    c. Shampoo your hair?   _____
II.   **Arising**
    a. Stand up from a straight chair without using your arms for support?_____

III. **Eating**
   a. Cut your meat?   ____
   b. Lift a full cup or glass to your mouth?   ____
IV. **Walking**
   a. Walk outdoors on flat ground?   ____
V. **Hygiene**
   a. Wash and dry your entire body?   ____
   b. Use the bathtub?   ____
   c. Turn faucets on and off?   ____
   d. Get on and off the toilet?   ____
VI. **Reach**
   a. Comb your hair?   ____
   b. Reach and get down a 5 lb. bag of sugar that is above
      your head?   ____
VII. **Grip**
   a. Open push-button car doors?   ____
   b. Open jars that have been previously opened?   ____
   c. Use a pen or pencil?   ____
VIII. **Activity**
   a. Drive a car?   ____
For reasons other than arthritis, I do not drive.   ___ Yes ___ No
   b. Run errands and shop?   ____

SOURCE: James F. Fries, Patricia Spitz, R. Guy Kraines, and Halsted Holman, "Measurement of Patient Outcome in Arthritis," *Arthritis & Rheumatism*, vol. 23, no. 2 (Feb. 1980). Reprinted with permission.

Managing Rheumatoid Arthritis

Rheumatoid arthritis cannot be cured, but it can be managed. As with diabetes and high blood pressure, you can maintain your health as much as possible through a combination of diet, exercise, medication, supplemental therapies, and regular checkups.

It is always good to be an active participant in your medical care, but this is especially true with rheumatoid arthritis. Because the disease varies and symptoms may come and go, your rheumatologist will rely on you to keep track of new developments, disease flares, and how you have responded to various therapies. You can use the Symptom Tracking Chart (Table 1 in chapter 4) to help keep track of symptoms.

Above all, remember that rheumatoid arthritis requires a multi-faceted treatment strategy. The exact combination of tactics will depend on your health, the severity of your disease, and your preferences.

Education and Support

Learning more about rheumatoid arthritis is the first step in becoming more empowered to cope with your disease and its treatments. Many studies also show that education and support help alleviate your pain and may reduce the number of times you visit your rheumatologist every year.

Your rheumatologist may have some brochures, videos, and fact sheets that will help you better understand the disease. If not, seek out a local support group, find the nearest chapter of The Arthritis Foundation, or contact one of the organizations listed in appendix A.

Diet and Exercise

If you have rheumatoid arthritis, you may lose your appetite. You might feel listless and not have the energy to get out and move. But to maintain your overall health and to help keep your symptoms under control, it's important to eat a well-balanced diet and exercise regularly and safely.

A healthy diet is one that includes all the nutrients we need to keep our bodies functioning well. This is especially important if you have rheumatoid arthritis because your body consumes more nutrients than normal when your symptoms flare.

Unfortunately, although a new "arthritis diet" seems to appear every week, there is no diet that will cure your disease. There is some evidence that eating foods high in omega-3 fatty acids, found in cold water fish such as mackerel, may make you feel better. And some people with rheumatoid arthritis find that certain foods don't agree with them. But then, that is true of everyone.

The best advice is the one your mother gave you growing up: Eat your fruits and vegetables and lay off the sweets. Try to eat less fat and more fruits and vegetables; less red meat and more fish. Try to consume low-calorie foods that will help you lose weight, which in turn decreases the pressure on your sore joints. Follow the guidelines of the FDA, which publishes the "food pyramid," about which foods to eat. And consider taking a multivitamin since some people with rheumatoid arthritis become deficient in certain vitamins (especially vitamin D, which helps maintain bones). You should also consider a calcium supplement (1,000 to 1,500 milligrams per day, depending on your age and any medications you are taking). For more information about the components of a healthy diet, see chapter 3.

Regular exercise is also important as long as it is done in a way that will protect your joints. If you are physically fit, you will be better able to cope with your disease. You will increase the range of motion in your joints, fight fatigue, strengthen muscles to provide better support to your joints, and improve your overall well-being.

The components of a good fitness plan include three major types of exercise:

1. Resistance exercises, which strengthen muscles and provide stronger support to your joints
2. Flexibility exercises, which improve your range of motion and reduce the risk of injury
3. Aerobic exercises, which improve the functioning of your heart and lungs and increase endurance

Since you want to protect your joints as much as possible, you might consider taking up sports like bicycling and swimming. And if you're experiencing a flare in symptoms or if your joints hurt before you even start, go easy on them. Try some gentle range-of-motion exercises to preserve mobility but otherwise rest your joints until the pain and inflammation subside.

Rest and Relaxation

There was a time when people with rheumatoid arthritis were advised to take to their beds. No longer. Too much inactivity can only make your joints stiffer and eventually might cause your muscles to weaken. The key is to balance healthy activity with periods of rest. Coping with the symptoms of rheumatoid arthritis can make you tired, so you may need to take "breaks" during the day. And if your symptoms are flaring, you might need more sleep than usual at night.

When your symptoms have subsided, you might be tempted to overdo things and end up exhausting yourself. Work with your rheumatologist and physical or occupational therapist to find the right balance between rest and activity. This may take some time, but it will be worth it. You will keep your joint inflammation under control and will feel more energetic.

Learning how to relax is also important if you want to keep your symptoms at bay. Stress can make any illness worse, and it can certainly aggravate the symptoms of rheumatoid arthritis. But stress is part of rheumatoid arthritis. There is physical stress placed on joints by the disease itself, and there is also emotional stress that comes from worrying about a chronic condition and the impact on your life.

Fortunately, you can reduce your stress levels. Relaxation tapes help some people; finding a support group helps others. And regular exercise—just getting yourself out and moving—will channel any tension and calm you down.

Joint Protection

Participating in sports like swimming and bicycling rather than running is one way to protect your joints, but you can adapt a number of other strategies to provide day-to-day protection.

Think about the way you use your joints during the day (you'll be surprised how often you use them) and think about ways to reduce any strain. For instance, use an electric can opener rather than a handheld one. Use your strong healthy joints instead, thereby protecting your weak or affected joints; for example, push open a door with your healthy shoulder rather than with your arthritic hand. For more advice about joint protection see chapter 10.

Many pharmacies sell assistive devices that may also help you. In the early stages of rheumatoid arthritis, your hands and feet may be weak and sore. Wedged insoles for shoes and ankle supports may make it easier to walk. Likewise, a splint for your lower arm, which will support your wrist joint so that it doesn't strain, will not only provide pain relief but also reduce damage to your wrist.

Physical and Occupational Therapy

Physical and occupational therapy will help you build muscle strength and recover range of motion in your affected joints, and are as essential as the other treatment strategies we've discussed. Rheumatoid arthritis requires a two-prong approach.

Exercise Tips

- Take a warm bath or shower before exercising; this will relax your muscles and reduce pain.
- If a particular joint is inflamed and sore, consider using an orthotic device to protect it (such as a splint to protect your wrist).
- To protect your back, you can sit in a chair while doing many range-of-motion exercises or hold on to the back of a chair.

Sample hand exercise to improve your ability to grasp objects:

1. Make a loose fist.
2. Bring your fists up to your shoulders, bending your arms at the elbows.
3. Lower your fists slowly.
4. Fan out your fingers, one at a time, so that they are straight.
5. Repeat.

Sample foot and ankle flexibility exercise:

1. Stand behind a chair with your feet on the floor.
2. Holding on to the chair for support, position your feet in a v.
3. Slowly bend your knees and crouch down, keeping your back straight.
4. Hold for a count of 3 (longer if you can).
5. Stand up slowly.
6. Repeat.

If you are experiencing a flare of symptoms and your joints are swollen, red, and warm to the touch, go easy on exercise. Try to move your joint slowly through its full range of motion. If it's too sore to move on its own, take your hand and gently move it passively. This will prevent tissue scarring and stiffness that can occur if you don't move the joint. Do this two or three times a day for short periods.

Once the flare subsides, begin doing active range-of-motion exercises for each joint. Then strengthen the muscles by doing isometric exercises, which involve tensing and releasing the muscles without actually moving your joint. You may find it easier to do this in the shower or even under the covers when your joints are warm. See chapter 10 for examples of exercises.

Medication Strategies

A dramatic change in the treatment of rheumatoid arthritis took place in the 1990s as rheumatologists learned more about the nature of the disease and scientists discovered new medications to treat it. The result is that the old approach of starting off with mild medications and holding the stronger ones in reserve until the disease had advanced has been turned on its head.

Disease-modifying anti-rheumatic drugs (DMARDs), once used as a treatment of last resort after others had failed, are now recommended as first treatments along with non-steroidal anti-inflammatory drugs, which reduce pain and inflammation. This new approach reflects the growing awareness among rheumatologists that early DMARD treatment may prevent or reduce disability in rheumatoid arthritis.

As the pace of laboratory discovery continues, additional drugs have been added to the arsenal available to fight rheumatoid arthritis. Some of these drugs have been approved by the FDA for use in rheumatoid arthritis, and others are in the pipeline. Now more than ever it is important to be well versed in treatment options so that you can discuss them with your rheumatologist.

Your rheumatologist will likely recommend an initial therapeutic strategy, then ask you to monitor what happens. Keep track of the medications you take, other factors such as diet and exercise, and how you respond. The initial strategy may be revised as time goes on, depending on how you feel and how the disease progresses.

In about 10 percent of patients, rheumatoid arthritis goes into remission, generally during the first year or two after onset. If you are one of these lucky few, your rheumatologist will ask to see you periodically to determine if the disease has begun to flare again.

More often, people with rheumatoid arthritis have a chronic condition that requires some type of treatment regimen for the rest of their lives. You should discuss medication options with your healthcare provider and rheumatologist before making any decisions.

Non-steroidal Anti-inflammatory Drugs (NSAIDs)

As previously discussed, NSAIDs, such as ibuprofen and *Aleve,* can reduce inflammation when prescribed in higher doses and are effective in combating pain, but they do nothing to slow the progression of rheumatoid arthritis. For this reason your healthcare provider may recommend that you take them while you wait for other medications to become effective. For more information about the risks and benefits of NSAIDs, see chapter 5.

COX-2 Inhibitors

If you are at high risk for suffering gastrointestinal upset or stomach bleeding, or if you have had an ulcer that has since healed, your rheumatologist may prescribe one of the new COX-2 inhibitors, which can alleviate pain and seem to have fewer side effects than aspirin or other NSAIDs.

COX-2 inhibitors act only on the COX-2 enzyme, which causes pain and inflammation, while ignoring COX-1, which is involved in protecting the lining of the stomach. In doing so, COX-2 inhibitors appear to reduce the most common side effect of NSAIDs: gastrointestinal disorders.

The FDA has approved one COX-2 inhibitor for the treatment of rheumatoid arthritis: celecoxib, marketed under the brand name

Celebrex. A second, rofecoxib, marketed as *Vioxx,* has been approved for osteoarthritis but not yet for rheumatoid arthritis (it is currently under study). Other COX-2 inhibitors are in various stages of development. See chapter 5 for more information.

DMARDs: The Current Backbone of Treatment

Disease-modifying anti-rheumatic drugs, or DMARDs, slow the progress of rheumatoid arthritis. In some cases they may even halt the disease. It is often unclear if the disease has gone into remission on its own or because of treatment with DMARDs.

Many DMARDs, such as hydroxycholoroquine, gold salts, and azathioprine, have been around for years. Others, such as methotrexate, have been used to treat rheumatoid arthritis only since the mid-1980s.

Although much remains unknown about their mechanisms of action, DMARDs appear to inhibit inflammation of the joint, which in turn may slow the destruction of joints and cartilage.

DMARDs sometimes take weeks or months to take effect, and they do not interfere with basic pain mechanisms, as NSAIDs and analgesics do. And yet DMARDs do eventually reduce pain, sometimes more effectively than NSAIDs, because they act on the underlying problem of inflammation that causes pain in the first place. For all these reasons, DMARDs are generally used in conjunction with NSAID treatment.

See Table 9, Disease-modifying Anti-rheumatic Drugs, for more detailed information about generic and brand names and dosages.

DMARDs Generally Tried First

HYDROXYCHLOROQUINE

As is sometimes the case in medicine, a medication that is effective at treating one type of disease will also prove helpful at treating another. That is the case with hydroxychloroquine, which was originally developed as an anti-malarial medication. In the 1950s and

Table 9. **Disease-modifying Anti-rheumatic Drugs**

Drug (Generic Name)	Drug (Common Brand Names)	Standard Doses
Auranofin (oral gold)	*Ridaura*	6–9 mg/day in 1 or 2 doses
Azathioprine	*Imuran*	50–150 mg/day in 1 to 3 doses, based on body weight
Cyclosporine	*Neoral* *Sandimmune*	100–400 mg/day in 2 doses; dose is based on body weight
Gold salts	*Aurolate* *Solganol*	10 mg in a single dose the first week; 25 mg the following week; then 25–50 mg/week; frequency may be reduced after several months
Hydroxychloroquine	*Plaquenil*	200–400 mg/day in 1 or 2 doses
Leflunomide	*Arava*	10–20 mg/day in single dose
Methotrexate	*Rheumatrex*	7.5–25 mg/week either as a single dose or split up over a 24-hour period; may also be given as an injection
Sulfasalazine	*Azulfidine*	2 to 3 gr/day in 2 to 4 doses
Biological Response Modifiers		
Etanercept	*Enbrel*	25 mg 2 times per week, given by injection
Infliximab	*Remicade*	3 mg/kg intravenously every 8 weeks

Data derived from The Arthritis Foundation ("Drug Guide," *Arthritis Today,* Jul./Aug. 1999, pp. 36–39).

1960s clinical studies showed that it was also effective in treating rheumatoid arthritis.

Hydroxychloroquine tends to cause less toxicity or side effects than other DMARDs but may take anywhere from three to six months to take effect and even up to twelve months to reach maximum therapeutic value. It also may remain in the body for as many as five years after the last pill is taken.

In rare cases hydroxychloroquine may damage the macula, the fine-tuning area of your eye. This condition is very rare and generally occurs at doses higher than those required to treat rheumatoid arthritis. To reduce toxicity you will receive a dose based on your body weight. To further reduce the chance that you will suffer eye damage, we recommend that you see an ophthalmologist once or twice a year. The ophthalmologist may discover problems before you even notice them. If eye toxicity should occur, the drug will be discontinued, and generally your eye problems will not get worse. Hydroxychloroquine has been known to cause light sensitivity, nausea, and diarrhea in some people.

METHOTREXATE

Methotrexate was first developed as a treatment for leukemia and at lower doses for psoriasis, a skin disorder that results in patches of inflamed red skin. Its usefulness for the treatment of joint disease was discovered when rheumatologists noticed that people with inflammatory arthritis who received methotrexate for psoriasis showed improvements in their joints as well as their skin. In 1988 the FDA approved it for use in treating rheumatoid arthritis.

Methotrexate is the most frequently prescribed DMARD. It acts faster than older DMARDs and takes effect in three to four weeks once the optimal dose is determined.

Although the exact mechanism of action is unclear, methotrexate appears to act on certain immune system cells and reduce inflammation. (For more information about how the immune system goes awry in this disease, see chapter 2.)

Methotrexate is highly effective; however, it may cause side effects, including mouth irritation, nausea, diarrhea, and vomiting. Methotrexate also inhibits a person's ability to metabolize and use folic acid, a vitamin that helps regulate cell growth. Some of these effects can be countered by lowering the dose or by taking folic acid, without interfering with methotrexate's beneficial effects. Check with your rheumatologist.

Less often, methotrexate can cause liver damage. If you drink alcohol regularly, you may be at increased risk of damaging your

liver while on methotrexate, so it is best to stop drinking while taking this medication. In rare cases methotrexate can damage lungs.
If you develop a cough or find yourself short of breath while taking
this drug, contact your rheumatologist.

Because methotrexate is excreted by the kidneys, it should not
be used by those who are on dialysis or have suffered kidney damage. If you have mild kidney problems, consult your rheumatologist
about whether this medication is right for you.

While taking methotrexate you should not receive a live vaccine
(including the chickenpox; oral polio; and measles, mumps, and
rubella vaccines) without first talking to your rheumatologist.

**If you are pregnant or planning to have children, do not take
methotrexate. This medication may cause birth defects if
taken at the time of conception or during pregnancy. If you
stop taking methotrexate for one menstrual cycle before trying to conceive, you will avoid this risk. If you want to
become pregnant or already are, it is important to discuss
safe medication strategies with your rheumatologist. (For
more information on arthritis and pregnancy, see chapter 12.)**

To avoid unwanted side effects, your rheumatologist will perform a blood test before prescribing the medication. If you do start
taking methotrexate, you will undergo regular blood tests to ensure
that you are suffering no adverse effects.

Methotrexate should be taken only once a week. If you take it
more often, you risk side effects. Try to take it on the same day each
week. Some people split the doses, such as Sunday morning and
Sunday night.

SULFASALAZINE

This drug is used to treat certain bowel diseases, such as colitis
and Crohn's disease. It is most often used in the treatment of milder
forms of rheumatoid arthritis and appears to work like methotrexate—by suppressing parts of the immune system.

Because sulfasalazine combines salicylates and sulfa, it is not recommended for those allergic to sulfa compounds. The medication also causes some side effects, including gastrointestinal distress, nausea, vomiting, rash, and headaches. In rare instances it may affect the white blood cell count. Decreased sperm count can occur but normalizes when the drug is discontinued. Routine lab monitoring is required.

Other DMARDs

AZATHIOPRINE

This DMARD functions as an immunosuppressive (it is known to inhibit the immune system). Originally used to prevent rejection of transplanted organs, azathioprine was later used as a treatment for people with rheumatoid arthritis who did not respond to conventional treatments. As with other DMARDs, azathioprine is delayed in its action; it can take three months for any benefit to be noticed and often takes six months or longer to become fully effective.

This medication may result in a number of side effects, including nausea. As an immunosuppressant it reduces your body's ability to protect itself against infections, so it is best to call your rheumatologist if you develop a fever or chills. Before taking the medication, make sure you know all the risks and benefits for you personally.

CYCLOSPORINE

Like azathioprine, cyclosporine is a type of immunosuppressant that is used to help prevent the rejection of a transplanted organ.

Cyclosporine can cause side effects ranging from excessive hair growth and elevated blood pressure to more serious problems like kidney dysfunction. It is not recommended for those who already have high blood pressure or kidney or liver disease. This medication is usually reserved for those who do not respond to other DMARDs.

GOLD SALTS

Gold salts reduce disease activity, although exactly how they do so is not known. Since other drugs were introduced, gold salts are not used as frequently as they were years ago. When used, gold salts are given as pills or as injections.

Side effects such as rash, mouth irritation, and diarrhea may occur if you take gold salts. Blood and urine are monitored on a regular basis for toxicity.

DMARD Combination Therapy

Although individual DMARDs are often effective in slowing the progression of rheumatoid arthritis, they may be even more effective when combined. This approach is similar to that used in the treatment of cancer where different forms of chemotherapy are combined to maximize effect. Combinations include the following: methotrexate and cyclosporine; methotrexate and anti-TNF therapy; and methotrexate combined with hydroxychloroquine and sulfasalazine.

Studies comparing DMARD combinations to individual DMARD treatment have found that they offer increased benefits to patients while not increasing side effects or toxicity. The combinations decrease swelling in the joints, increase mobility, and improve overall health. The benefits are especially evident after one year of treatment, in particular for triple combination therapy.

Corticosteroids

Corticosteroids are synthetic versions of hormones naturally produced by the adrenal glands, located near your kidneys. They are often mistaken for but are not at all similar to the type of steroids that some athletes use to build their muscles and increase their competitive edge.

Corticosteroids provide fast and powerful reduction of inflammation for many people with rheumatoid arthritis. As such, corticosteroid injections are used in the treatment of rheumatoid arthritis, and are particularly helpful if you are having a flare-up in symptoms.

Injections of corticosteroids provide relief and reduce inflammation and pain while waiting for DMARDs to become effective. When given in oral or pill form, corticosteroids suppress inflammation throughout your body. Prednisone is the most frequently used corticosteroid for treatment of rheumatoid arthritis, but there are many others; see Table 10.

TABLE 10. **Corticosteroids Used to Treat Rheumatoid Arthritis**

Drug (Generic Name)	Common Brand Names
Cortisone	*Cortone Acetate*
Dexamethasone	*Decadron, Hexadrol*
Hydrocortisone	*Cortef, Hydrocortone*
Methylprednisolone	*Medrol*
Prednisolone	*Prelone*
Prednisolone sodium phosphate (liquid only)	*Pediapred*
Prednisone	*Deltasone, Orasone, Prednicen-M, Sterapred*

Data derived from The Arthritis Foundation ("Drug Guide," *Arthritis Today*, Jul./Aug. 1999, pp. 36–39).

Corticosteroids have been used to treat rheumatoid arthritis since the 1950s. The initial effect was so impressive that some healthcare providers regarded these treatments as a possible cure. That notion passed quickly, however. If administered in too high a dose or for prolonged periods of time, they can cause a number of side effects, including weight gain, osteoporosis, cataracts, hypertension, blood sugar elevation, and increased susceptibility to infections and bruises. In the years since corticosteroids were first introduced, we have learned how better to marshal the therapeutic benefits of steroids without exposing patients to their dangerous side effects. This includes using lower doses.

Although specifics may vary, all corticosteroids appear to have similar mechanisms of action. They impair the production of potentially destructive inflammatory cells in the joint while preventing others from reaching the area. This helps explain why corticosteroids are so helpful. But they also decrease production of collagen, a central building block for many tissues in our bodies, including cartilage, and inhibit the absorption of calcium, which could increase the rate of bone destruction.

In general, the higher the dose of a corticosteroid, the greater its effect on reducing inflammation and the faster it acts—but the greater chance that it will cause side effects. As a result, your rheumatologist will likely weigh the need for rapid action against your ability to tolerate the side effects. And whatever oral medication is used, the dose will likely be tapered as time goes on to reduce long-term effects such as bone thinning (osteoporosis) and cataracts.

Before giving injections directly into your joint, your rheumatologist will first remove excess fluid from the joint area. The benefit of these injections is temporary pain relief, but too many injections may actually damage your joints. For this reason injections should be given only three or four times a year into the same joint. In addition, corticosteroids should be used in conjunction with DMARDs and not as a sole treatment.

Tetracyclines

Medications in the tetracycline family have potential for the treatment of rheumatoid arthritis. Long valued for their ability to fight infections, this family of medications is receiving renewed appreciation and investigation.

Tetracyclines do not cause many side effects and are relatively easy to take. A number of studies in animals as well as people show that they may also inhibit certain immune system cells and chemicals that destroy cartilage early on in rheumatoid arthritis.

Doxycycline and minocycline, types of tetracycline that have been used to treat acne, are being studied in osteoarthritis and rheumatoid arthritis.

The New Medicines

Many medications used to treat rheumatoid arthritis were originally developed for other diseases such as cancer, malaria, and psoriasis. While effective, none has produced what rheumatologists and sufferers alike are searching for: long-term remission and even a cure. And many cause side effects that are distressing and sometimes health-threatening.

The latest wave of research is yielding medications that may solve some of these problems. Some are biological response modifiers that have been impressive in terms of treatment, literally changing the immune system response that goes overboard in rheumatoid arthritis by targeting specific immune cells. Others improve existing treatments or introduce whole new approaches in the management of rheumatoid arthritis.

Biological Response Modifiers

Also known as biological agents, biological response modifiers home in on specific immune system cells that destroy joints without affecting other aspects of immunity, thus avoiding some of the side effects and risks of more traditional medications.

Because of the way they target the immune system cells, biological response modifiers are sometimes referred to as "heat-guided missiles" or "smart bombs." They are generating much excitement in the field not only because they work so well, but because they are opening the door to a new era in the treatment of rheumatoid arthritis.

The FDA has approved two biological response modifiers for the treatment of rheumatoid arthritis: etanercept (brand name *Enbrel*) and infliximab (brand name *Remicade*). Additional biologic agents are in the pipeline and may be approved for use in the next few years.

ETANERCEPT (*ENBREL*)

Marketed under the brand name *Enbrel*, etanercept targets tumor necrosis factor (TNF), which plays a major role in making joints swollen and painful. TNF is a cytokine, a type of protein that helps regulate the functions of many cells, including those involved in inflammation. In healthy people the levels of TNF circulating in the bloodstream is kept in balance, but if you have rheumatoid arthritis, the level of TNF increases dramatically, leading to swelling and pain and contributing to other destructive aspects of rheumatoid arthritis.

Etanercept is a synthetic protein that essentially acts as a decoy for the TNF circulating in your bloodstream. It binds with TNF molecules, thereby preventing them from penetrating the cells to continue the process of inflammation. By capturing TNF in this way, etanercept supplements the body's naturally occurring TNF regulators so that they are not so overwhelmed.

Etanercept must be injected; there is no pill form. You will receive the medication in powdered form and will be taught how to turn it into a solution. Twice a week you (or a partner) inject the medication into your thigh, abdomen, or upper arm. (Your rheumatologist or nurse will show you how.)

In between injections, store the powdered form of the medication in the refrigerator (not the freezer). You can also premix a solution, but this should not be stored in the refrigerator for more than six hours. Etanercept contains a protein that can decompose if stored at room temperature, and the drug may no longer be effective. Discuss these issues with your healthcare provider and follow the instructions on taking this medication carefully.

Benefits of etanercept. Etanercept is used in people who have active rheumatoid arthritis and have not significantly improved after treatment with DMARDs. Your rheumatologist may also recommend that it be used before other therapies are tried.

For many the results are dramatic. In clinical studies about 60 to 70 percent of those taking etanercept reported a lessening in pain and joint swelling. Etanercept boosts energy levels and shortens the amount of morning stiffness. You may find that you can get out of bed more easily, reach objects on shelves without difficulty, and have the stamina to play with your children. In fact, etanercept improves aspects of life across the board as measured in health status instruments—everything from appetite to physical activity.

The drug acts quickly, in as little as two weeks, although it may take three months to feel the full effect. Studies that have been ongoing for three years show that the drug continues to work as long as you take it, and X rays show that it slows damage to the joint.

Etanercept also appears to boost the effectiveness of traditional DMARD therapy. Adding etanercept to standard methotrexate therapy, for instance, resulted in a 75 percent improvement in the number of tender joints—almost double that provided to people who took methotrexate alone. No doubt other combinations will be tested as additional biological modifiers are discovered.

Risks and side effects. The most common side effects of etanercept are related to the injection. Some people report redness, pain, itching, and swelling.

You should not take etanercept if you have an active or chronic infection, as it reduces TNF levels in your bloodstream, which appears to be important in the defense against certain infections. You should also read the ingredients carefully; don't take etanercept if you have an allergy to any of them. And while taking etanercept, you should not receive a live vaccine (such as the chickenpox; oral polio; or measles, mumps, and rubella vaccines) without first talking with your healthcare provider or rheumatologist.

Costs and other issues. Etanercept is more expensive than many other medications: about $250 per week, or $12,000 per year. Some insurance plans may not cover it. See Table 11, Cost of Medications.

TABLE 11. **Costs of Most Frequently Prescribed Medications Used in Treating Rheumatoid Arthritis**

Disease-modifying Anti-rheumatic Drugs (DMARDs)

Drug (Brand Name/ Generic Name)	Standard Dose	Average National Retail Price	Estimated Yearly Cost
Arava	1 tablet/day (20 mg)	$243.87	$2,926.44
Azulfidine	4 tablets/day (500 mg)	$46.38	$556.56
Plaquenil/ hydroxychloroquine	2 tablets/day (200 mg)	$82.15/ $52.74	$985.80/ $632.88
Rheumatrex/ methotrexate	3 tablets/day (2.5 mg)	$57.24/ $26.51	$686.88/ $318.12
Sandimmune	1 tablet/day (100 mg)	$193.08	$2,316.96

Data derived from The Arthritis Foundation (*Arthritis Today*, Sept./Oct. 1999), p. 43, based on information from D. P. Hamacher & Associates, Inc., and Merck Co., Inc.

Biological Response Modifiers

Drug (Brand Name)	Estimated Cost
Enbrel	$1,000 month, or $12,000/year (twice-weekly injections)
Remicade	$1,222 for each 8-week dose, or about $8,000/ year plus the cost of infusions (actual dose will depend on body weight)

Data derived from The Arthritis Foundation (*Arthritis Today*, Jan./Feb. 2000, pp. 40–41).

Because etanercept was only recently approved by the FDA, further studies are under way to evaluate its effectiveness and safety.

INFLIXIMAB (REMICADE)

Another biological agent, infliximab (brand name *Remicade*), also targets tumor necrosis factor (TNF) but in a different way from etanercept. Rather than acting as a decoy, infliximab uses a monoclonal antibody that hunts down TNF and neutralizes it so that it has no effect.

Imfliximab was originally approved by the FDA for treating Crohn's disease, a chronic inflammatory disease that affects the gastrointestinal tract. In 1999 it was approved for use in rheumatoid arthritis.

Infliximab is administered intravenously by a healthcare professional. It takes about two hours to receive the IV dose, which depends on body weight. During the initial period you will receive three IV doses over the course of six weeks. Then you will shift to a maintenance dose received every other month. In the first year you should expect about eight infusions; thereafter you will receive about six doses per year.

This medication is given in conjunction with methotrexate, discussed above.

Benefits of imfliximab. The FDA approved infliximab for use by people whose rheumatoid arthritis has not responded well to methotrexate alone. Early studies show that adding infliximab to the treatment regimen significantly improves a range of symptoms—often within two weeks—although it can take several months to enjoy the full effect. Joint swelling and pain decreased, mobility and overall health increased, and functional ability, as measured by a health assessment instrument, improved as well. You may find you can dress yourself with less hassle, walk without pain, and reach and grab for things much more easily.

Nearly one in three people taking infliximab along with methotrexate had at least a 50 percent improvement, compared with one in twenty taking methotrexate alone. And X rays show that infliximab decreases damage to the joint.

Risks and side effects. Rarely do people develop reactions to the infusions. Overall, however, fewer side effects are reported with infliximab than with some of the more traditional drugs.

You should not take infliximab if you have an active or chronic infection or if you develop one while on the medication. Talk with your rheumatologist. Because infliximab reduces levels of TNF (an immune system component), you may be less able to defend yourself against certain infections.

Costs and other issues. Like many new medications, infliximab is relatively expensive, costing from $8,000 to $10,000 a year (see Table 11). Check your health insurance policy to see if this type of medication is covered and if there are any limits or exclusions. And talk with your healthcare provider and rheumatologist if you have any questions.

Because infliximab has only recently been approved for the treatment of rheumatoid arthritis, long-term studies about its safety and effectiveness continue. Talk with your rheumatologist about the most recent studies.

More Research on Biological Response Modifiers

Etanercept and infliximab may be only the beginning. Additional immune system targets for biological agents are now being studied. Interleukin-1 (IL-1), which is also involved in inflammation, immune system response, and joint destruction, is one such target. Inhibitors of IL-1 may help reduce the joint destruction in rheumatoid arthritis.

Investigators are also looking into combining inhibitors of IL-1 with inhibitors of TNF, such as etanercept and infliximab, and other targets as well. More research needs to be done, but this is a promising area of investigation right now.

LEFLUNOMIDE (ARAVA)

Leflunomide, marketed under the brand name Arava, is a type of immunosuppressant that belongs to the family of DMARDs. Although its exact action in rheumatoid arthritis is unknown, this new medication appears to work by inhibiting immune cells that promote inflammation in joints.

In early clinical trials leflunomide worked as well as the more standard DMARDs, methotrexate and sulfasalazine. As such, it may provide another option for you if you are currently using DMARDs as part of your treatment regimen.

This medication alleviates pain and swelling, and reduces the total number of tender joints. Studies have shown that it slows the progression of the disease. Leflunomide must be prescribed; it should be taken once a day and at the same time every day. It may take a month before you notice any benefit.

The most common side effects of leflunomide are abdominal pain, diarrhea, rash, and hair loss (but these end when the medication is discontinued).

While taking leflunomide, you will have your blood tested regularly to monitor for drug toxicity.

Leflunomide can cause birth defects. It also remains in the body long after the last pill was taken. If you are taking the medication currently but want to become pregnant, speak with your rheumatologist. He or she can best advise how to discontinue the drug and can recommend a treatment to eliminate it from your body, making it safe to conceive. While waiting, make sure you and your partner are using birth control.

The Prosorba Column: A Blood-filtering Device

If you have moderate to severe rheumatoid arthritis and have not benefited from treatment with one or more DMARDs, another option is the Prosorba column, a blood-filtering device approved for use in March 1999 by the FDA.

The Prosorba column functions much like a kidney dialysis machine. You are connected to the device, your blood is withdrawn through a tube, filtered through the column, removing certain substances involved in rheumatoid arthritis, and then returned to your bloodstream.

The procedure takes about two hours, and is usually done once a week for twelve weeks. It can be done on an outpatient basis. Clinical studies showed that it generally took all twelve treatments before people noticed any benefit.

Side effects most commonly reported are chills, mild fever, nausea, and joint pain (similar to that of a flu) for a day or two after treatment. Other side effects include headache, anemia, sore throat, abdominal pain, rash, and dizziness.

Complementary Therapies

Because rheumatoid arthritis affects you on so many different levels, you may feel better if you add one or more complementary therapies to your treatment regimen. Evening primrose oil and fish oil supplements are particularly noteworthy because they have been shown to decrease pain and swelling in joints.

Before using complementary therapies, discuss them with your healthcare provider or rheumatologist who may relate precautions you are not aware of. For instance, massage may sound like a gentle therapy, but a massage therapist who is not familiar with rheumatoid arthritis may inadvertently press too hard on joints already damaged or inflamed.

The FDA does not regulate herbal and vitamin supplements the same as it does drugs. (Herbs and vitamins are considered "dietary" supplements, and Congress exempted them from regulation in 1994.) This means it is important to become a skeptical consumer. Just because a product's package claims certain benefits does not mean they are guaranteed. And the quality and active ingredients contained in various supplements may vary depending on the manufacturer.

So ask a lot of questions, learn more about the complementary approaches, and discuss them with your healthcare provider. For more information about complementary therapies see chapter 11.

Surgery

If you have suffered severe damage to one or more joints because of your rheumatoid arthritis, your rheumatologist may recommend that you see an orthopedic surgeon. Several types of surgery may benefit you and allow you to regain function. Surgery can indeed be a miracle. For more details see chapter 13.

CHAPTER 8

Taking Charge of Other Types of Arthritis

IT WOULD be impossible to discuss every form of arthritis in this book. What follows is a brief discussion of symptoms and treatments for the most common types of arthritis besides osteoarthritis and rheumatoid arthritis.

Inflammatory Arthritis

Ankylosing spondylitis and psoriatic arthritis are both forms of inflammatory arthritis. These conditions may accompany skin disorders such as psoriasis, inflammatory intestinal disorders like Crohn's disease, and other chronic disorders.

Ankylosing Spondylitis

The name *ankylosing spondylitis,* which is quite a mouthful to say, derives from the Greek for vertebra, *spondylos,* and inflammation, *itis.* The inability of a joint to move is called *ankylosis.* This type of arthritis affects the spinal column. Tendons and ligaments that attach muscles to the spine become inflamed, limiting movement and causing pain. If the disease progresses, vertebrae in the spinal column fuse and the back becomes rigid.

Ankylosing spondylitis affects men more often than women, typically developing between the ages of sixteen and thirty-five. Although the cause of the disease remains unknown, the genes associated with ankylosing spondylitis are inherited, so if you have family members with this type of arthritis, you are more at risk yourself. Fortunately, if the condition is diagnosed and treated early, you should be able to lead a normal life.

EARLY SYMPTOMS

Early signs of this disease are low back pain and stiffness that persist for months. Although backaches plague many people, you can distinguish the pain caused by ankylosing spondylitis in the following ways:

- The pain develops slowly over several weeks rather than coming on suddenly
- The pain persists for at least three months at a time, rather than coming and going in acute but short-lived bursts
- The stiffness and soreness appear early in the morning or after sitting for a long time, but improve after movement and exercise
- The symptoms appear at a relatively young age, typically the mid-twenties

Although ankylosing spondylitis affects your spine, you may first feel an ache in your buttocks or down the back of your thighs, as well as in your lower back. The pain may be worse on one side than on the other.

The parts of the spine affected are shown on page 167. Ankylosing spondylitis usually starts in the lowest part of the back, in the sacroiliac joints between the sacrum and the pelvis. For reasons that remain unclear, this part of the back becomes inflamed, causing pain. The bone begins to grow in an abnormal way, around the joint.

Feeling ill and fatigued is also common during the early stages of ankylosing spondylitis. Or you may feel depressed and lose weight without trying. These symptoms are similar to those experienced by people with rheumatoid arthritis and result, in part, from your inflammatory response, which takes a toll not only on your joints but also on the rest of your body.

AS THE DISEASE PROGRESSES

If ankylosing spondylitis is not diagnosed and treated early enough, it may progress. (A lucky few people will experience remission, as is the case for rheumatoid arthritis, but this is the exception rather than the rule.) Should your disease continue, new bone may form around the sacroiliac joints, eventually fusing the joints. Similar changes take place in the lower spine, and the vertebrae may begin to fuse.

The Spine

The spine is made up of 33 bones called vertebrae and is divided into 5 regions. Vertebrae of the sacrum and coccyx are fused and immobile. The remaining vertebrae provide the flexibility to bend, stretch, and lift.

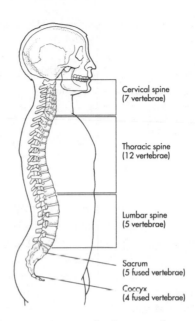

Cervical spine
(7 vertebrae)

Thoracic spine
(12 vertebrae)

Lumbar spine
(5 vertebrae)

Sacrum
(5 fused vertebrae)

Coccyx
(4 fused vertebrae)

If your ankylosing spondylitis progresses farther up the spine, you may find it harder to breathe or that it hurts when you breathe. You are experiencing these symptoms because the joints between your ribs and your spine are affected. Because your chest movement may become restricted, it is especially important that you don't smoke; that would further restrict your ability to breathe.

The disease may also begin to affect other joints in your body, typically the shoulders, hips, and knees. In addition, as many as 40 percent of people with ankylosing spondylitis develop a type of eye inflammation known as acute anterior uveitis. Symptoms include eye pain, sensitivity to light, excess tearing, and impaired vision. The condition can be treated with topical medications, or you may require oral corticosteroids. You can avoid long-term damage if the condition is diagnosed and treated early enough.

HOW ANKYLOSING SPONDYLITIS IS DIAGNOSED

If you suspect you might have ankylosing spondylitis, it is best to see a rheumatologist to find out for sure. An aching back can result from many conditions, including a slipped disk or muscle strain, as well as ankylosing spondylitis.

To determine what is causing your symptoms, your healthcare provider will take a medical history and do a physical examination. He or she may take an X ray of your spine and order an ESR test, which provides an indirect indicator of how "active" your disease is. (See chapter 7 for further discussion of the ESR test, which is also used in diagnosing rheumatoid arthritis.)

Treatment

There is no cure for ankylosing spondylitis, but there are multiple treatments available. In this type of arthritis as in the others, a multifaceted approach will bring about the best results.

There are several things you can do to help yourself. Although this will sound like advice you received growing up, it applies to ankylosing spondylitis: Get enough sleep, eat right, exercise, and stand up straight.

Because ankylosing spondylitis results in part from inflammation (a type of immune system response), you may find you feel tired and fatigued. Even if you don't, you should try to get enough sleep and avoid overly stressful activities. You need energy to cope with the symptoms and the resulting inflammation. Try to avoid overtime on your job and try not to overschedule your free time.

Diet is also easy to overlook. In inflammatory types of arthritis such as ankylosing spondylitis, you may lose your appetite, but it's important to eat well-balanced meals anyway so that you get the calories that are converted into energy. By eating right you'll improve your mood and energy levels. For more information about eating right, see chapter 3.

We should all exercise regularly—at least thirty minutes a day according to most health experts. But regular physical activity is especially important if you have ankylosing spondylitis. Since the disease can cause stiffness and immobility, you should focus on exercises that promote flexibility and mobility. A physical therapist can design your program, but see the sample exercises in chapter 3.

MAINTAINING GOOD POSTURE

Because this type of arthritis may result in vertebrae fusing, it is especially important to keep your spine straight at all times—at work, at home, and even while asleep. Otherwise, your spine may fuse in a curved position, and you will not be able to stand up straight again. (You may have seen someone walking in a hunched-over position. This could be the result of advanced ankylosing spondylitis that was never treated.)

To maintain good posture, the first thing to do is become more aware of how your back and upper torso feel when you are standing straight. Your shoulders are back, your chest thrust slightly forward, and your backside slightly outward. Your arms should dangle by the sides of your thighs, not in front of them.

Choose chairs that offer firm support and a straight back. Some people also find armrests comfortable. If you have an office job, try to take a five-minute break every hour; otherwise, you will become too stiff. The same applies to a long car drive. If you have a manufacturing or assembly job, try not to hunch over the work area.

Even at night you must try to protect your spine. Replace a mattress that sags with one that is firm; if you can't afford to, put a board under the part of the mattress where you sleep. Even a sheet of plywood will do. And don't use pillows; these force your head forward for as much as eight hours a night (or more if you sleep longer). That could result in your spine fusing in a forward position. You may find it comfortable to sleep without a pillow, or you may need a cervical pillow that supports the upper portion of your spine. Your physical therapist can advise you on which option would be best for you.

PHYSICAL THERAPY

Because maintaining mobility and good physical habits are so important in managing ankylosing spondylitis, your healthcare provider will probably suggest that you see a physical and/or occupational therapist. As discussed further in chapter 10, these professionals are skilled at teaching you how to protect your joints and strengthen your muscles so that you can continue living your life as you always have—or close to it.

Some people think physical therapy is a long, involved process, but it usually involves only one or two visits plus periodic returns for an assessment of how you're doing. Your physical or occupational therapist will design a home exercise program for you that you can continue on your own. Most provide handouts with illustrations to jog your memory.

Typically, a physical or occupational therapy consult will involve the following:

Learning more about your goals. You will be asked a series of questions, such as: What activities do you want to maintain? What activities have caused you the most pain? What do you do for a living? The answers to these questions will help the therapist focus on those issues that are of concern to you.

Assessment of current habits and challenges. Your physical or occupational therapist will take a look at how you hold yourself while sitting, walking, and standing. He or she will ask about your work and home environment: what kind of chairs you sit on, how much you move about, and what types of activities have been compromised since you began feeling pain. Because maintaining good posture is so important in the management of ankylosing spondylitis, your therapist will make recommendations about how you can improve your posture and might recommend exercises as well as adaptive equipment.

Don't be surprised if the therapist asks about activities you may not think much about, such as how you get dressed, how you bathe or wash yourself, how and where you drive, and how you hold the phone or type on a keyboard at work. All these mundane tasks affect your spine, and if you relearn some of them, you may find that your pain subsides and you feel better.

Exercises. In addition to making you more aware of how you sit, stand, walk and sleep, your physical therapist will show you how to improve all these activities. Simple exercises can improve your muscle tone, flexibility, and endurance. Exercises that stretch the trunk of your body—from your neck to your hips—are especially important to help improve your posture. Some of these exercises can be done standing up, others lying down. The emphasis will be on muscle extension to maintain flexibility. Your physical therapist may also recommend deep-breathing exercises to ensure that you can continue to expand your chest as much as possible. See chapter 10 for more about exercise.

Your physical or occupational therapist will also show you how to do hip and leg exercises designed to extend and stretch the muscles supporting the joints in the lower part of your body. These weight-bearing joints provide support for your whole body and can come under extra strain if your back hurts. By strengthening and extending these muscles you can counteract the damage. A deceptively simple exercise is to lie prone on the floor or a firm surface for as long as you can manage, up to a maximum of an hour. You may find that this gets easier as the muscles in your legs and hips loosen up. The therapist may also provide specific exercises for your shoulders to improve range of motion and muscle strength.

Swimming is an excellent all-around activity because it strengthens muscles and improves cardiovascular fitness without putting any strain on joints. But almost any physical activity you enjoy can help you become fit. Activities you should avoid include diving off a diving board (because you risk damaging your neck) and extended bicycle trips (because you are in one position for a long time).

Adaptive equipment. If your physical or occupational therapist thinks you need to do more to protect your joints or if your mobility has already been limited, he or she will recommend adaptive equipment and joint supports. For instance, elongated rearview mirrors that attach to your car's current rearview mirror will enable you to see blind spots while driving without turning to the right or left. To protect your neck from injury in the event of a car accident, make sure the head supports on the backs of seats are in the proper position.

Although your back may hurt, especially at the beginning of your physical therapy plan, your therapist probably will not suggest that you wear a brace or other type of supporting corset. If you wear these devices, your muscles may atrophy, and this would only worsen the situation. It is far better in the long run to strengthen your own inner assets—your muscles—to support your spine and the rest of your joints.

Medication Strategies

NSAIDs and COX-2 inhibitors may help alleviate your pain and inflammation, and other treatment options are available if these do not work for you.

NSAIDs. At low doses, NSAIDs relieve pain; at higher doses, they also reduce inflammation. (see chapter 5 for more information). The FDA has approved the following NSAIDs specifically for the treatment of ankylosing spondylitis:

- Diclofenac
- Indomethacin
- Naproxen
- Sulindac

See Table 12, FDA-Approved Non-steroidal Anti-inflammatory Drugs for Ankylosing Spondylitis. As always, check with your healthcare provider to see if this type of medication is appropriate for you.

COX-2 inhibitors. The FDA has not approved the use of COX-2 inhibitors specifically for ankylosing spondylitis, but your healthcare provider may suggest that you try using them to control pain. For more information about how they work, see chapter 5.

Few clinical studies have been done on other medications to prove whether they are effective for this type of arthritis. Drugs used to treat rheumatoid arthritis are also sometimes used to treat ankylosing spondylitis. These drugs are used in conjunction with the NSAIDs mentioned above, and include sulfasalazine, originally developed to treat inflammatory bowel disease, and methotrexate, used for psoriasis and rheumatoid arthritis.

Sulfasalazine has been studied the most and might be of benefit if you have just been diagnosed with ankylosing spondylitis or have not responded to other treatments. Some rheumatologists think sulfasalazine and methotrexate actually slow development of ankylosing spondylitis; they appear to be most effective in treating arthritis in joints other than the spine.

TABLE 12. **FDA-Approved Non-steroidal Anti-inflammatory Drugs for Ankylosing Spondylitis**

Drug (Generic Name)	Common Brand Names	Standard Dose
Short-acting		
Diclofenac potassium	Cataflam	100–200 mg/day in 3 or 4 doses
Diclofenac sodium	Voltaren	150–200 mg/day in 3 or 4 doses
Diclofenac sodium with misoprostol	Arthrotec	100–200 mg/day in 2 to 4 doses *Note: These doses apply only to the diclofenac portion, the dosage of misoprostol will vary depending on the strength of the pill.*
Long-acting		
Indomethacin	Indocin	50–200 mg/day in 2 to 4 doses
Naproxen	Naprosyn	500–1,500 mg/day in 2 doses
	Naprelan Naprosyn-E	750 mg or 1,000 mg/day in a single dose
Sulindac	Clinoril	300–400 mg/day in 2 doses

Data derived from The Arthritis Foundation (*Arthritis Today*, July/Aug. 1999, pp. 30–32).

Complementary Therapies

You may also find it helpful to add complementary therapies to your treatment plan. To deal with pain, for instance, you can apply heat or a warm compress. A nice hot shower is one way to bathe your back in warm water. A heating pad may also work wonders.

Some people also find massage helpful, especially in soothing aching muscles and encouraging relaxation. And although most types of massages are safe, your spine is vulnerable when you have ankylosing spondylitis and may already have developed some damage. For that reason you should talk with your healthcare provider before getting one for the first time. He or she may be able to provide a referral to a particular massage therapist or at least let you know what to avoid.

Surgical Treatments

Should ankylosing spondylitis progress to the point where your spine has become fused and/or bent, your healthcare provider may suggest surgery to correct the problem. This type of surgery is risky, however, since damage to the nerves in the spinal cord can result in paralysis. Before deciding to undergo surgery, give the matter a great deal of thought about the risks as well as the benefits—and get a second opinion.

If the disease spreads to joints other than your spine, damaging the cartilage and other structures of the joint, your healthcare provider may recommend joint replacement surgery. Typically, this type of surgery, which involves replacing the damaged parts of the joint with artificial joints (usually made of hard plastic), is performed on hips and knees. Although any surgery should be undertaken with caution, this operation may help restore movement in joints that have suffered extensive and irreversible damage.

Psoriatic Arthritis

Psoriasis is a skin disease in which scaly red and white patches develop. About 5 percent of people with psoriasis develop psoriatic arthritis in which the joints become swollen and sore. There is no link between the pattern or extent of psoriasis and the eventual development of arthritis. If you have a severe case of psoriasis with extensive scaly patches, you are no more likely to develop arthritis than someone with more limited psoriasis.

The symptoms of psoriatic arthritis differ from one person to the next, but there are some recognizable patterns:

- In about half of those affected, a joint will become arthritic on one side of the body but not the other (that is, not both knees or both wrists).
- In about one in four people, the same joint on both sides of the body is affected (that is, both knees).
- In about one out of fifteen people, the fingers and toes are most affected.
- In about one out of twenty people, the disease will distort the shape of the joint.

Like the skin disease it is associated with, psoriatic arthritis is characterized by symptoms that flare and then subside. Different joints also may be involved from one time to the next. And like ankylosing spondylitis and other types of inflammatory arthritis, other problems such as eye inflammation can develop.

Fortunately, if you have psoriatic arthritis, you have a number of treatment options to choose from, and even more therapies may be discovered in the years ahead.

What You Can Do for Yourself

There is no cure for psoriatic arthritis, but it can be managed. And the first step in managing it is to pay better attention to the fundamentals of good health: a balanced diet, regular exercise, and sufficient rest. For more information see chapter 3.

Beyond that, look for advice from your physical and/or occupational therapist, who can help evaluate how to adjust your daily activities and schedule to conserve energy and protect your joints. In general, your physical or occupational therapist will recommend the same strategies as for rheumatoid arthritis. See chapter 7 for more details.

However, there are a few differences in approach with psoriatic arthritis. If you have a severe form of this disease, your muscles may contract suddenly and painfully. One way to prevent this is to pay attention to flexibility exercises, which lengthen and loosen muscles and increase your range of motion. (See chapter 10 for more information about flexibility exercises.)

If muscle spasms become a problem, your physical or occupational therapist may recommend that you wear a splint or some other brace. Hand and ankle splints, for instance, can prevent feet and hands from contracting. Because psoriasis may make it difficult to wear braces or other supports (since your skin will itch and feel uncomfortable), your physical or occupational therapist may suggest that you wear a cotton glove or lining in addition to the particular brace or splint recommended. (Cotton is best. A lining made of nylon or another artificial material will only worsen the situation because it doesn't allow the skin to "breathe.")

If your feet are affected, look for shoes with a lot of room in the toe area in case your toes swell. Soft inserts for the sole and ankle supports or orthotics may also provide some extra support when you need it.

Finally, if your joints are inflamed, try a cold pack to reduce the swelling. If your joints are sore, moist heat may help.

Treatment Strategies

We don't know what causes psoriatic arthritis and are only beginning to understand how this disease begins and progresses. For that reason we tend to use treatments that have proven successful in other types of inflammatory arthritis.

Your healthcare provider will do a physical examination, take blood tests, and may take X rays to determine which of your joints are affected, how badly they are damaged, whether they are inflamed, and how extensive your skin disease is.

Psoriatic arthritis requires a team approach, and your healthcare provider may consult with both a rheumatologist, who can advise about your arthritis, and a dermatologist, who can recommend treatment of the skin disease. Your joints may improve when your skin does.

First options. Your healthcare provider may first recommend that you take COX-2 inhibitors or NSAIDs to control pain and inflammation. For more information about these treatments, see chapter 5.

Corticosteroid injections. These synthetic versions of hormones produced naturally by the adrenal glands can be injected directly into an inflamed joint. They produce relatively quick and effective relief of pain and inflammation. For more information about this strategy see chapter 6.

Additional options. If NSAIDs or COX-2 inhibitors do not relieve your symptoms, your rheumatologist may recommend adding other treatments, the disease-modifying antirheumatic drugs, or DMARDs. These medications, which are used to treat rheumatoid arthritis, appear to slow the progress of inflammatory arthritis.

Generally speaking, methotrexate may be the most effective medication for this type of arthritis. This medication was actually first developed to treat psoriasis. Later researchers found that it effectively treats rheumatoid arthritis and other inflammatory forms of arthritis. Methotrexate is one of the most commonly prescribed DMARDs, and a number of studies have shown it to be one of the most effective. Methotrexate takes about four to six weeks to take effect, but once the benefit is achieved, it can remain effective for years. Liver toxicity is the major concern with this drug in psoriasis.

Other options besides methotrexate include gold salts and sulfasalazine. There is no cookie-cutter rule for the strategy, however, because every person responds differently to drugs and experiences different types of side effects.

A newer medication, etanercept *(Enbrel)*, has recently been studied in psoriatic arthritis, and results have been encouraging for both the improvement of the arthritis and the skin disease. Studies on the use of leflunomide *(Arava)* and infliximab *(Remicade)* for psoriatic arthritis are also in progress. See chapter 7 for more information about DMARDs and these newer medications.

Complementary Therapies

Those who have psoriatic arthritis may feel they have been doubly cursed—by psoriasis and arthritis. For that reason it may be helpful to supplement treatment with complementary therapies.

Psoriasis tends to worsen when you are feeling stressed. Likewise, the pain of your arthritis may also be more intense at those times. For that reason you should try to find a way to relax. This may be as simple as finding a quiet spot each day and listening to

music or a relaxation tape. Or you can take a class in yoga or meditation (which are getting easier and easier to find). You may also find
that an occasional massage provides relief—as long as your psoriasis
is not acting up in the same area.

If your skin is acting up, particularly around the affected joints,
you may be feeling particularly miserable. (Itching and aching
together may seem like too much to handle!) You might try to apply
a soothing topical cream to the area. Many people find lotions and
creams that contain aloe helpful. (This product comes from the aloe
plant and is also used to soothe burns and dry, chapped skin.)

To provide extra relief from pain and inflammation, you may also
want to take a zinc supplement. Zinc is one of the minerals we need
every day to be healthy, and there is some early evidence that a zinc
supplement helps reduce swelling and promotes overall well-being
in people who have psoriatic arthritis or rheumatoid arthritis. Talk
with your healthcare provider before taking zinc or any other supplement because of possible interactions with other medications
you are taking.

Polymyalgia Rheumatica

Polymyalgia rheumatica (PMR) causes stiffness, pain, and limited
mobility in the neck, shoulders, upper arms, lower back, hips, or
thighs. If you suspect you have PMR, it's important to see a healthcare provider to find out for sure. People with PMR are at
increased risk of developing temporal arteritis, a type of inflammation that affects the arteries located between the scalp and the eyes.
Temporal arteritis, which is easily treated with higher doses of cor-
tisone, could lead to blindness if not treated.

This type of arthritis usually develops in people over sixty years
of age, although it can start as early as forty-five. The disease can
come on suddenly or so slowly it is barely noticed. Symptoms
include morning stiffness and fatigue, and a general feeling of listlessness. You may also lose weight without trying, run a low-grade
fever, or have a severe headache with sharp pains, or tenderness in

your scalp. You may experience disturbances in your vision or even lose your sight because of diminished blood flow to the optic nerve through inflamed arteries. Not surprisingly, you may also feel depressed and confused.

Although its symptoms resemble other types of arthritis, PMR is unique in that it tends to flare up for a temporary period, usually two or three years, and then subside so completely that the disease seems to go away.

Medication Strategies

Treatment for PMR can last anywhere from one month to two years. It is impossible for a healthcare provider to predict the exact duration in advance.

If you have a mild form of PMR, your healthcare provider may prescribe a non-steroidal anti-inflammatory drug (NSAID). If you have not responded to NSAIDs, you may receive low doses of corticosteroids, synthetic versions of natural hormones produced by the adrenal glands. There is often a dramatic response to low-dose steroids (15 milligrams per day or less of prednisone). Corticosteroids are effective at reducing pain and inflammation but can cause side effects that include weight gain, hypertension, and increased risk for osteoporosis. For more information on NSAIDs and corticosteroids, see chapter 5.

If you have PMR, the condition may interfere with your day-to-day activities until you are treated. Such corticosteroids as low-dose prednisone are generally quite successful in controlling symptoms. You will need to deal with the side effects of medication, however.

If your healthcare provider does prescribe corticosteroids, you should also take supplemental calcium and vitamin D to reduce the risk of osteoporosis. Regular exercise also helps prevent bone loss. (See chapter 3 for more information on the fundamentals of a good diet and basic fitness plan.)

If you feel anxious or worried about your condition, you may want to use some of the complementary therapies described in greater detail in chapter 11. In particular, relaxation techniques and meditation may help lower your blood pressure and help you cope better.

Arthritis in Children

Raising a child is challenging even under the best of circumstances, but if your child has arthritis, you have even more to contend with. Thanks to new treatments and a growing array of support services, however, your child should be able to grow up normally and reach his or her full potential.

In children with arthritis, as in adults, early intervention improves outcomes, and that intervention is likely to consist of exercise and physical therapy as well as medication. The goal is to control your child's arthritis and enable him or her to develop as normally as possible.

Arthritis is rare in children, but when it does occur, it comes in many guises—some similar to that seen in adults and some unique to children. There are childhood forms of rheumatoid arthritis, ankylosing spondylitis, reactive arthritis, and psoriatic arthritis. The most common type of arthritis seen in children is juvenile rheumatoid arthritis (JRA).

Juvenile Rheumatoid Arthritis

Juvenile rheumatoid arthritis (JRA) is a type of autoimmune disorder in which your child's immune system begins attacking his or her joints. (For an explanation of how this happens, see chapter 7.) As in the adult form, JRA causes different types of symptoms in different children. These multiple subtypes include:

- Systemic disease, which is associated with high fever and rash; it affects various parts of the body in addition to joints
- Polyarticular, which affects multiple joints at once
- Pauciarticular, which affects only a few joints

The cause of this disease remains unknown. As is typical of autoimmune diseases, JRA affects about four times as many girls as boys.

SYMPTOMS

Symptoms of JRA appear most often between the ages of two and five but can occur in children at any age. If your child has JRA, you may notice that one or more joints have become swollen or warm. He or she may move stiffly, especially when first getting up in the morning, or may stumble or limp. After moving around a bit, the joints loosen up. Or your child may whine or cry and tell you it hurts (although, especially young children may not be able to say exactly where it hurts). Or you may notice that your child is irritable and has changed play habits.

Other symptoms affect other parts of the body besides the joints. You may notice that your child's lymph nodes in the neck or armpits are swollen. He or she may develop a fever that fluctuates from normal to over 103 degrees Fahrenheit at night. A red rash may appear on the arms, legs, abdomen, and chest. Appetite and weight loss may also occur.

Children with JRA may be at increased risk for eye inflammation. Untreated, this could lead to loss of vision. If your child is diagnosed with JRA or even if it is suspected, it is important to make an appointment for an evaluation by an ophthalmologist.

HOW ARTHRITIS IS DIAGNOSED IN CHILDREN

If you suspect that your child has JRA, make an appointment with a pediatrician, who will ask you about the symptoms you've observed, do a physical examination, examining your child's joints for signs of inflammation, and possibly order blood tests to exclude other illnesses and to monitor your child's overall health status.

If your child has JRA, also consult from then on with a rheumatologist, a specialist in diseases of the muscles, bones, and joints. There are also pediatric rheumatologists who specialize in the care of children with arthritis. Referrals to such specialists are absolutely essential.

Ask for referrals to other healthcare providers, such as physical or occupational therapists and nutritionists, to ensure that your child grows up as healthy as possible.

Your Child's Healthcare Team

Pediatrician This primary care doctor is trained to recognize a broad array of illnesses and conditions in a child.

Pediatric rheumatologist This specialist is a pediatrician who has had advanced training in the care of children with diseases affecting the joints, muscles, and connective tissues such as skin and blood vessels.

Nurse specialist or nurse practitioner These nurses receive advanced training in various fields, including arthritis and orthopedics.

Occupational therapist This professional works with your child to find ways to reduce the wear and tear on joints during daily activities at school or at home. Special attention is paid to joints in the hands and arms.

Pharmacist This professional can explain how your child's medications work and what side effects might develop—and, if possible, how to lessen them.

Physical therapist This health professional works with your child to strengthen muscles and improve mobility.

Also essential:

Dentist A skilled practitioner who treats diseases of the teeth and gums is necessary because the medication your child takes may affect oral health. Your child's dentist should also know about your child's arthritis and medications before performing certain invasive procedures that require anesthesia or sedation.

Ophthalmologist This physician treats eye diseases. Since eye inflammation is associated with JRA, frequent eye exams are necessary to help prevent serious problems from developing.

Orthopedic surgeon This physician is able to perform specialized surgery to repair joints if necessary.

Arthritis remains a relatively rare problem in children, and few pediatricians have seen enough children with this condition to have the perspective of a specialist. Moreover, new insights into JRA are being gained each year (sometimes, it seems, each month). To ensure that your child gets the best care possible, insist that a specialist be part of the healthcare team.

WHAT YOU CAN DO TO HELP YOUR CHILD

All parents want their child to stay healthy. If your child has arthritis, you may already feel defeated, but children with arthritis can learn to work around their condition just as children with diabetes do. It is just a matter of learning what to avoid and what to encourage. Here is how you can help:

Educate yourself about JRA. One of the most vexing things about JRA is that it can flare and subside, and that symptoms are so varied. The condition may be chronic, meaning your child could have it for the rest of his or her life. All too often parents feel overwhelmed, depressed, and confused.

One way to feel more in control is to learn as much as you can about your child's JRA. The best place to start is with your child's rheumatologist. Ask for any brochures and pamphlets that may be available. Another good place to start is with the Arthritis Foundation, a nonprofit organization that produces a slew of educational materials, pamphlets, and videos. The American Juvenile Arthritis Organization, a council of the Arthritis Foundation, sponsors regional conferences that will enable you to meet the parents of other children and will also provide an opportunity for your child to meet and interact with other children with JRA.

Last, but nowadays in no way least, is the Internet. A number of reputable sites—some sponsored by the government, others by nonprofit organizations, and still others by universities—provide good information (see appendix A).

Encourage your child to eat healthy foods. Diet is certainly a key factor in helping your child become as healthy as possible. During childhood and adolescence, your child is growing so fast that he or she needs a well-balanced diet to provide the proper nutrition. As discussed in chapter 3, a good diet consists of meat, fresh fruits and vegetables, dairy products, nuts, and grains.

If your daughter has JRA, make sure she consumes enough calcium every day (although this is something all girls should do). Calcium helps build and strengthen bones and prevent osteoporosis later on. She should consume 1,300 milligrams of calcium every day, about the amount in four cups of milk or three cartons of yogurt.

Encourage your child to play and exercise. Some well-intentioned parents who have children with JRA try to protect their joints by limiting their activities, but regular exercise actually benefits the child in a number of ways. Studies have shown that exercise decreases pain, improves function (and avoids disability later on), and decreases a child's need for medication—not to mention that it will make him or her feel better, to feel like "one of the kids."

Why? As mentioned in chapter 2, our understanding of how arthritis develops and how it can be managed has changed in the past few years. We now understand that muscles play a big role in protecting and supporting the joints. That is why exercise is so crucial: it strengthens and builds a child's muscles. Regular exercise also improves a child's well-being, providing a boost to metabolism and immune system functioning.

But if your child is in pain, he or she may not want to exercise. And some activities should be avoided. For that reason it is best to consult a physical and/or occupational therapist early on to determine the best activities for your child. For instance, if you have a young child, certain toys will encourage movement and play in spite of low energy levels. Rolling a ball back and forth is a good and safe game for young children; just make sure the ball is lightweight. (Basketballs, for instance, may be too heavy for a child with JRA.) Tricycles and bicycles are also good choices since they enable a child to exercise muscles without putting extra strain on sore joints.

As your child grows older, encourage him or her to take up swimming and biking. Even hiking is fine, as long as your child isn't carrying a heavy backpack and keeps a reasonable pace.

What to avoid? High-impact sports (such as basketball and football) and jumping on a trampoline will only aggravate your child's arthritis. He or she should also try to avoid sustained repetitive motion such as typing on a computer keyboard for extended periods, or playing video games that require users to move joysticks or their thumbs back and forth again and again.

Use physical and occupational therapy. Although all exercise is important, there may be times when your child should do specific exercises. For instance, if joints become inflamed, it's best to help rotate the joint gently through its complete range of motion. This will prevent a joint from becoming overly stiff.

To alleviate pain and relax the muscles, either a cold pack or warm bath or wrap will help (as it does with adults). Show your child how to pack ice in a towel, or use a hot water bottle, to provide a sense of control over the situation. (If your child is young, you may want to buy a gel pack in the pharmacy to avoid messes.)

If a particular joint is acting up or causing continual pain, ask your child's pediatrician or physical or occupational therapist about a splint. These help keep your child's joint in alignment, reducing pain and inflammation. Knee and wrist splints, which keep the joint extended, are commonly used.

Advocate for your child in school. Your child has JRA but is just as bright and full of potential as any other child and may require only some reasonable accommodations in the classroom. To ensure that your child gets a good education in spite of having JRA, it's best to work with your child's school administrators and teachers from the very beginning. Your child may need special seating or permission to get up and stretch periodically or help with taking medications during the course of a school day. Working with appropriate school personnel should result in an approach that works for all concerned.

No child wants to feel different from others, and it is likely that your child will experience some problems with other children. The best approach is to encourage your child to talk about upsetting events and ways to handle the problem. If your child continues to have difficulty in dealing with classmates, speak with the teacher.

Be forewarned that you may need to educate these educators about JRA! Your child's teacher may never have had a child with JRA in his or her class before. (Hence the importance of educating yourself first.) Most people are reasonable and will provide accommodations once the issue is explained. If not, remember that the Americans with Disabilities Act—and most state education boards—insist that reasonable accommodations be made in educating a child with special needs. Remind your child's teacher of this, and if all else fails, approach the principal or superintendent.

In high school, different challenges emerge. Teenage years are never easy on anyone, but your child may feel particularly stressed and embarrassed about arthritis. A social worker or psychologist can help your child (and the whole family) learn ways to cope with JRA.

After high school comes college or a vocation. This raises whole new issues. If your child applies to college, evaluate potential schools carefully—not only for the types of academic programs that are offered but also for the type of services provided to students with special needs. Also look at the campus itself: Will your child be able to navigate it? Are there too many hills? Are the buildings so far apart that it will be difficult just going from a dormitory to a classroom? Are there medical facilities on campus? Where is the nearest hospital off campus? How far away is the college in case your child needs you?

If your child decides to go directly from high school into a job, you may want to consult with a school guidance counselor about vocational resources in your community. In particular, many vocational rehabilitation programs—which receive state and federal funds—help people with disabilities develop job skills and find work. If your child qualifies, this will help make the transition to the world of work.

Or perhaps your child will be able to find work without assistance. If so, he or she should follow commonsense precautions: avoid jobs that involve repetitive motion, high impact, or a lot of stress. If the job is sedentary, your child should take breaks to stretch and move around. See chapter 3 for more tips about protecting joints.

TREATMENT STRATEGIES

As with adults who have rheumatoid arthritis, the goal when treating children is to alleviate symptoms such as pain and inflammation while trying to slow the progression of the disease. But children face several challenges that adults do not when it comes to medication. Clinical studies to evaluate the effectiveness of new drugs are generally done in adults first, and there are few long-term studies, which look at a range of health indicators, about how outcome relates to a given treatment strategy in children. It is important to provide information about your child's symptoms and response to medication to your child's healthcare provider, who will then make adjustments to therapy as needed.

Aspirin. Long the mainstay of treatment for JRA, aspirin came under a cloud in the 1980s when its use in children was associated with the development of Reye's syndrome, a severe and sometimes fatal condition that begins as a mild illness but can lead to swelling of the brain, convulsions, and even coma.

But aspirin should not be dismissed out of hand. It comes in a number of different forms, including enteric-coated to avoid stomach problems and liquid preparations that may be easier for your child to take than pills. Aspirin may still be appropriate if your child has already had chickenpox and has not been exposed to an influenza infection.

To avoid problems, be alert to such side effects as:

* Abdominal pain, stomach upset, or diarrhea
* Ringing in the ears (tinnitus) or other hearing loss
* Changes in behavior
* Bruising
* Nose bleeds

Stomach upset is the most common. To lessen the chances of this happening, give the aspirin to your child with food (at the beginning of a meal) or give an enteric-coated pill.

COX-2 inhibitors. These are currently being studied in children, but as yet there are no data about their effectiveness. The FDA has not approved COX-2 inhibitors for use in children.

NSAIDs. For more information about these medications that reduce pain and inflammation, see chapter 5. Two NSAIDs, tolmetin and naproxen, have received FDA approval for use in children. Several others are routinely used. Table 13 includes typical doses for these medications.

Table 13. NSAIDs Typically Used to Treat JRA

Doses of drugs for children are determined by body weight (typically milligrams per kilogram, although your healthcare provider can explain how many milligrams per pound).

Drug	Typical Dose
Aspirin	75–100 mg/kg/day
Ibuprofen	30–40 mg/kg/day
Indomethacin	2–4 mg/kg/day
Naproxen	10–15 mg/kg/day
Tolmetin	20–35 mg/kg/day

Adapted from Bernhard Singsen and Carlos Rose, "Juvenile Rheumatoid Arthritis and the Pediatric Spondyloarthropathies," in Michael Weisman and Michael Weinblatt, eds., *Treatment of the Rheumatic Diseases* (Philadelphia: W.B. Saunders Co., 1995), p. 220.

Because NSAIDs increase stomach acid levels, you should give your child the medication before the start of a meal to lessen the chance of stomach upset. Since NSAIDs may cause kidney damage, your child should undergo a renal function test before taking an NSAID.

Some children experience side effects such as dizziness, mild headaches, ringing in the ears, confusion, mood changes, and problems concentrating. Others also suffer fatigue and vision problems. There is no evidence that NSAID use increases the chance of your child's developing Reye's syndrome. Contact your healthcare provider if your child experiences any unusual symptoms while taking an NSAID.

DMARDs. Disease-modifying antirheumatic drugs appear to slow the progression of rheumatoid arthritis in children as well as adults. (See chapter 7 for more information.) Here is a brief description of each of the DMARDs used for children.

Methotrexate is one of the most commonly prescribed DMARDs in adults. A clinical study published in 1986 showed it was effective for JRA as well, and it has emerged as the treatment of choice for many rheumatologists.

Methotrexate reduces inflammation by inhibiting certain types of immune system cells. It therefore seems to slow disease progression by halting the assault on joints and bones. It is appropriate to use for a child with JRA who has the disease in multiple joints and has not responded well to NSAID treatment, but it may also be used if the arthritis is so severe that the child has limited motion in an affected joint, has suffered bone growth abnormalities, or has an eye inflammation (anterior uveitis) that has not responded to other treatments.

Methotrexate is generally well tolerated by children, but side effects similar to those in adults can occur such as mouth irritation, nausea, diarrhea, and vomiting. For this reason a blood test is performed every four to eight weeks to monitor toxicity. Talk with your child's rheumatologist about how to minimize side effects.

A child who is taking methotrexate should not receive a live vaccine (which includes the chicken pox, oral polio, and MMR vaccines) before you have talked with a pediatrician or rheumatologist.

Hydroxychloroquine was originally developed to fight malaria but may be effective for a child when combined with other medications. Some studies suggest that this medication is as effective as gold salts, but causes fewer side effects.

In rare cases hydroxychloroquine may damage the macula, the fine-tuning area of the eye. Although this condition is very rare, your child should see an ophthalmologist on a regular basis in order to detect problems before they become apparent. If eye toxicity should occur, the drug is stopped, and generally the eye problems do not get worse. Hydroxychloroquine has caused light sensitivity, nausea, and diarrhea in some people.

Etanercept: a biological response modifier. Healthcare providers have long searched for medications that are more specific in their actions, affecting only the disease process. Recently, research has yielded a number of biological response modifiers that target specific immune system cells involved in rheumatoid arthritis. While they are not "magic bullets," biological response modifiers have proven effective in the treatment of adult rheumatoid arthritis (see chapter 7). One of these biological response modifiers, etanercept, marketed under the brand name *Enbrel,* has been approved by the FDA for use in children. Etanercept targets tumor necrosis factor (TNF), which plays a major role in swollen and painful joints.

In healthy people the level of TNF circulating in the bloodstream is kept in balance, but in JRA the level of TNF increases dramatically, leading to swelling and pain and contributing to other destructive aspects of rheumatoid arthritis. Etanercept is a synthetic protein that essentially acts as a decoy for the TNF circulating in the bloodstream.

Etanercept must be injected; there is no pill form. You must inject the medication into your child's thigh, abdomen, or upper arm twice a week. (Your child's rheumatologist or nurse can show you how.) In between injections the medication should be stored in the refrigerator. Etanercept contains a protein that will decompose if stored at room temperature, and the drug will not be effective.

Benefits. Early studies show that etanercept is very effective for children with JRA who have not responded to other medications. In one study more than 70 percent of children taking etanercept noticed an improvement in symptoms. For one out of three the improvement was so dramatic that their activities returned to normal.

The drug acts quickly—in as little as two weeks, although it may take three months to feel the full effect.

Risks and side effects. Your child should not take etanercept if he or she has an active or chronic infection. This medication reduces TNF levels in the bloodstream, which may be important in your child's defense against certain infections. And while taking etanercept, your child should not receive a live vaccine (such as for chicken pox, oral polio, or MMR) unless you have first talked with his or her pediatrician or rheumatologist.

The most common side effects are redness, pain, itching, and swelling at the site of the injection. These generally subside as the injections are continued.

Because etanercept was only recently approved by the FDA, questions remain about long-term safety. Further studies are under way to evaluate the effectiveness and safety of this drug.

OTHER MEDICATION STRATEGIES

Corticosteroids. There are times when corticosteroids are useful. Because they are relatively fast acting, corticosteroids taken in pill form can be used if your child has just been diagnosed with severe JRA. This medication acts as a therapeutic bridge, buying time until other medications become effective. Injections of corticosteroids into the affected joints may help restore movement, especially if the joint or joints have not responded to NSAID treatment. Intravenous doses are sometimes required to treat other symptoms of JRA, such as high fever, symptom flares, or inflammation of the heart and/or lungs.

Because corticosteroids may stunt growth and development, they should be given sparingly and in the lowest doses possible.

Immunosuppressive medications. This group of medications is used only as a last resort if your child has not responded to NSAIDs or DMARDs and is facing life-threatening complications from JRA. Immunosuppressive drugs may make your child more vulnerable to infections and infertility, and may even increase the chance of developing cancer as an adult.

Surgery. If treatment with medication is not effective, surgery may be necessary to correct the damage caused by JRA. In this event NSAID treatment is stopped three or four days before the actual surgery, especially if significant bleeding is expected. (If NSAID use is suspended, your rheumatologist may recommend temporary use of corticosteroids to keep disease activity in check.) As always, communicate with your child's rheumatologist and surgeon ahead of time.

There are many surgical options for children, including total joint replacement. For more details on surgery, see chapter 13.

Infectious Arthritis

This type of joint disease is caused by an invading organism. The infectious agent may travel from an open wound near the joint or through the bloodstream as a result of an infection somewhere else in the body.

The faster a diagnosis is made and treatment begins, the better the chances of recovery without suffering debilitating arthritis. Therapy generally involves antibiotics that destroy the infectious agent. If the arthritis has already progressed, other treatments may be required.

Infectious arthritis can develop as a complication of chickenpox, rubella, mumps, rheumatic fever, or gonorrhea. It can also be caused by microorganisms such as those that cause Lyme disease, tuberculosis, strep throat, influenza, bacterial endocarditis (a form of heart inflammation), and hepatitis (an inflammation of the liver).

Whatever the source of infection, the joint becomes warm to the touch as well as swollen and painful, possibly accompanied by fever and chills. If these symptoms occur after contracting one of the infectious diseases mentioned above, contact your healthcare provider. To determine the infectious agent responsible for your symptoms, your healthcare provider will remove synovial fluid from the affected joint or joints and culture it in the laboratory.

Lyme disease is probably the best-known type of infectious arthritis today. It has become the most common vector-borne illness in the United States. It is transmitted from one host to another by means of a tick. This disease will be explored in greater detail in the pages that follow.

Lyme Disease

Most people are disgusted by ticks, those tiny eight-legged insects that attach themselves to skin and feed on blood. Now people have reason to fear them as well because certain types of ticks carry the bacteria that causes Lyme disease.

Although the symptoms of Lyme disease were first identified in Europe in 1913, they were first reported in the United States in 1975 in Lyme, Connecticut, which gave the condition its name. The disease received a lot of attention with the explosion of the deer population in the mid- to late 1970s as more and more cases were reported.

Ticks inhabit grassy, woodland areas. The type of ticks that cause Lyme disease, notably the deer tick and the Lone Star tick, are most prevalent in the Northeast, upper Midwest, and far West, although cases have been reported in other parts of the country. People may come into contact with ticks when mowing the lawn, hiking, or even walking. The family dog may also transport ticks into the house.

Lyme disease is caused by a bacterium known as *Borrelia burgdorferi*, which is transmitted to the bloodstream once a tick bites you. Initially, the bite may escape notice since the tick is small (sometimes no bigger than a poppy seed), and the bite may appear only as a small red dot. Sometimes the reddened area will expand and measure several inches across. A hallmark sign of Lyme disease is the so-called bull's-eye rash, a red circle with clear skin in the middle, but an infected person may never have this kind of rash.

Symptoms. In its earliest stages, the symptoms of Lyme disease are subtle and may mimic other diseases. Fever, fatigue, muscle aches, and headache may be the first signs; they typically occur a few days or weeks after infection. A rash may also develop in the first few days after infection. This rash can last for a few hours or several weeks; it can be small or diffuse. Although the bull's-eye rash is associated with Lyme disease, other rashes may develop as well and may be mistaken for hives, eczema, sunburn, poison ivy, or mosquito bites.

Additional symptoms include:

• Painful and swollen joints, usually the knees or other large joints

- Difficulty chewing
- Frequent and painful urination
- Cough, asthma, pneumonia, and other respiratory infections
- Ear pain, hearing loss, ringing in the ears
- Eye inflammation, light sensitivity, conjunctivitis, blurred vision
- Sore throat, difficulty swallowing
- Burning, tingling, or prickling sensations; loss of coordination
- Dizziness, palpitations, light-headedness
- Mood swings, inability to concentrate, loss of memory
- Disabling heart failure and permanent nerve damage (in the most severe cases)

Symptoms may also be elusive, flaring for a week or so at a time and then disappearing. Small wonder that Lyme disease has been called the "great imitator."

Some people may not even know they are infected. The disease may play itself out in two or three years and leave no permanent damage even without treatment. But about 60 percent of people who contract Lyme disease and do not get treatment develop arthritis. Because it is impossible to predict which course the disease will take, you should consult your healthcare provider if you think you have been infected.

Diagnosis. Your healthcare provider will determine if you have Lyme disease after asking about your symptoms, analyzing the results of a preliminary blood test, and learning more about how and where you may have been infected. The two biggest clues are where you live and a reddish rash on your skin that may signify a tick bite. If your town is known to be in an area infected with ticks, your healthcare provider may be more likely to recommend treatment.

If all this sounds like detective work, it is. There are no direct tests for Lyme disease. The FDA has approved two blood tests to determine whether antibodies to *Borrelia burgdorferi*, the bacteria that causes Lyme disease, are present. (One can be analyzed in your healthcare provider's office; the other must be sent out to a laboratory.) But both tests are inexact, especially in the early stages of the disease.

If you are suffering the symptoms of Lyme disease–induced arthritis, your healthcare provider may also analyze your blood test for other signs, including an elevated "sed rate," which provides an indirect measure of inflammation and can be used to determine how active your arthritis is.

Treatment Strategies. Antibiotics are usually the first line of treatment for Lyme disease in its earliest stage. Generally, antibiotic treatment will continue for several weeks in pill form or intravenously. If the disease has progressed, additional antibiotics may be needed to fight the infection or an NSAID to control pain and inflammation. It can take as long as three months for antibiotic treatment to work.

If your Lyme disease has caused arthritis that has not responded to the initial dose of antibiotics, see a rheumatologist. He or she may try a different type of antibiotic or prescribe hydroxychloroquine, a disease-modifying antirheumatic drug (DMARD) originally developed to treat malaria. For more information about DMARDs, see chapter 7.

If you have already suffered joint damage and no other treatment works, your rheumatologist may recommend that you undergo a synovectomy, an operation to remove the diseased part of the joint membrane.

How to Avoid Getting Lyme Disease

Fortunately, there are ways to avoid contracting Lyme disease. These include the following simple precautions anytime you go outdoors, especially if you live in an area known to have a lot of ticks:

- Avoid tick-infested areas, especially from May through August. Such areas include woods and places with high grass and brush.
- Wear long-sleeved shirts when outside gardening or mowing. Pull socks up over long pants, creating a barrier that insects cannot penetrate.

- Wear light-colored clothing so that you can see the ticks more easily.
- Consider using insect and tick repellents on your body or clothing, but read the directions carefully and understand that no repellent is a guarantee against a tick bite.
- If you are hiking, try to stay on a path and avoid brush.
- If you are outside for a prolonged period, examine any exposed skin every few hours.
- Once inside, check your skin all over, especially skin folds such as under the arms, behind the ears, behind the knees, and between fingers and toes.
- Check other common areas ticks might hide, including the belly button, neck, hairline, and top of head.
- Take a shower after outdoor activities and wash the areas mentioned above; ticks may wash off if they have not yet firmly attached themselves.
- If you find a tick, remove it with tweezers. Do not try to remove it with your fingers or light a match and place it near the tick or dab with alcohol or petroleum jelly. These techniques could actually end up transmitting the bacteria to you.

Lyme disease vaccines

One vaccine for Lyme disease has been approved by the FDA, and others are in the pipeline. The vaccine *LYMErix* reduces the risk of becoming infected with Lyme disease. It is recommended if you live in a high-risk area, spend a lot of time outdoors, or have arthritis from a previous Lyme disease infection. But it isn't foolproof. Even when given exactly as instructed, the vaccine protects only four out of five people. (In addition the same ticks that carry the Lyme disease bacteria also carry other nasty infections.) And all of the vaccine's side effects are not yet known.

LYMErix must be given in three doses over the course of a year. The first and second doses are given a month apart, and the final dose is given one year after the first. They should be timed to coincide with the beginning of tick season—in April in the northeastern

United States. (The FDA is currently considering a proposal to compress the timetable for the shots.)

The FDA has not yet approved the medication for use in children under age fifteen or adults over age seventy. Still, the vaccine represents a promising step forward in trying to prevent Lyme disease in the first place.

Other Rheumatic Diseases

Gout

Gout develops when uric acid, a waste product, accumulates in the joints. Normally uric acid dissolves in the bloodstream and is excreted in urination. A person with gout either makes too much uric acid or is unable to excrete it properly. As a result, the uric acid forms crystals that settle in the joints and cause inflammation, resulting in sudden jabs of pain, soreness, redness, and swelling in the joints. Gout generally affects one joint at a time, most often the big toe, ankle, knee, foot, hand, wrist, or elbow.

Occasionally multiple joints can be affected, and sometimes the uric acid deposits show under the skin as bumps. These deposits can be seen most often on the arms and legs.

TREATMENT OF EARLY DISEASE

Gout is one of the better understood inflammatory diseases, and effective treatments are available. Unlike other fields in arthritis, where healthcare providers have become more aggressive in their treatment strategies and begin treatment early, in gout the trend has been the opposite: more conservative treatment first, followed by a period of watchful waiting to see if other attacks occur. The reason is that you may have one bout of symptoms and never experience a recurrence. Or you may experience a relapse, but it can take months or even years, and in the meantime you do not need medication.

For a first case of gout, treatment involves the following:

Rest. Resting your inflamed joint is important because putting pressure on it will only exacerbate inflammation. If you have an attack of gout in your feet, it's best to elevate the affected foot and take it easy until the inflammation subsides. If the attack is in your knee, rest and elevation may help, as well as a splint that provides support to your joint so that your muscles don't have to strain.

Gout in your hands or elbows may make it impossible to move the affected area until the attack subsides. Placing your arm on a pillow may help or use a splint to support your joints until the inflammation goes away.

Diet. Gout is the only type of arthritis that clearly responds to a change in diet. The condition develops when uric acid builds up in your bloodstream. Although we all make uric acid naturally, we make more of it when we eat foods that contain purines, substances found in meat and certain types of seafoods and vegetables. One of the best ways to avoid further attacks of gout is to stop consuming or consume much less of the following foods:

Alcohol	Meat
Anchovies	Mushrooms
Asparagus	Peas
Cauliflower	Poultry
Dried beans	Sardines
Herring	Scallops
Mackerel	Spinach

Your healthcare provider will likely recommend that you drink more fluids and avoid diuretics such as coffee that dehydrate you. Drinking more fluids (especially water) will help flush uric acid out of your body. Although the FDA recommends that everyone drink about two quarts of water every day, if you have gout you should try to drink even more—as much as three quarts a day. And avoid alcohol. Not only does it dehydrate you, but it also raises the level of uric acid in your blood.

NSAID treatment. If pain and inflammation persist or if the condition has already advanced, your healthcare provider will likely prescribe a non-steroidal anti-inflammatory drug to control pain and inflammation. Generally speaking, the strategy in treating gout is to begin with a higher dose while the attack is severe and then lower the dose to maintain the effect. For more information about NSAIDs, see chapter 5.

Corticosteroids. Synthetic versions of a hormone naturally produced by the adrenal glands, corticosteroids offer effective and relatively fast relief from pain and inflammation—but they have side effects ranging from weight gain to increased risk of osteoporosis. These need to be weighed against their benefits.

Your healthcare provider may inject a corticosteroid directly into your joint if you are suffering acute pain. These medications are also given in pill form or injected into a muscle to affect other parts of the body. This systemic approach is used when gout affects more than one joint or when you have not responded to other treatments.

Colchicine. Derived from the saffron plant, colchicine was first used to treat gout in the seventh century. For years colchicine was the mainstay for the treatment of gout, but as more effective and less toxic medications were discovered, it fell out of favor. (About half of people who take colchicine experience side effects, mostly vomiting and diarrhea.) But there are still times when it is appropriate to use colchicine, and it is safe if used according to established guidelines. The medication is useful in preventing additional acute attacks and is often used in combination with corticosteroids.

PREVENTING FURTHER ATTACKS

The goal in treating gout is to prevent further attacks. Your healthcare provider may recommend that you discontinue certain medications such as diuretics that increase your uric acid level. Simple lifestyle changes such as diet can help prevent new crystals from forming. You should also lose weight since every extra pound places more pressure on your joints.

You can undertake these changes once you have brought the initial symptoms under control. Your healthcare provider may also advise that you continue taking NSAIDs or colchicine for months or years depending on your particular situation, to ensure the problem does not recur.

Allopurinol (brand names *Lopurin* and *Zyloprim*) is used to prevent further gout attacks. This medication was originally developed for the treatment of cancer but was subsequently found to reduce uric acid levels. It is also useful in cases of chronic gout. This medication may take months to achieve its full therapeutic effect.

Sometimes an attack of gout may occur after starting allopurinol; changes in uric acid levels are the reason. It is important not to stop taking allopurinol if you have an attack; it is important to take this medication every day for the rest of your life.

Additional medications include those that increase the excretion of uric acid in the urine, such as probenecid and sulfinpyrazone. These are effective for most people but are not advised if you have kidney disease. To minimize the risk of side effects, drink plenty of liquids.

CHAPTER 9

Coping with Conditions That Mimic Arthritis

SOME MEDICAL conditions feel like arthritis but are not diseases of the joint. Such conditions include bursitis, tendinitis, and fibromyalgia. These disorders cause pain, stiffness, and sometimes an overall feeling of being sick—but they affect the muscles and tendons, not the joints themselves.

The good news for people with these disorders is that they don't cause joint destruction. So if you can alleviate the symptoms, life should return to normal, and your joints will remain as healthy as they were before.

Bursitis

Jane was a multitasker. She often cradled the phone between her ear and her shoulder while leaning on her elbow and leafing through files or reaching across for the computer mouse. She kept meaning to get a speaker phone but never quite got around to it. Plus she always felt like she had to shout into it just to be heard. But lately she noticed her left elbow had developed a painful lump, making it impossible to lean on. What on earth was this?

Any bony protrusion on your body, such as your knee, shoulder, or elbow, is covered by a tiny fluid-filled sac, or bursa. We each have about 150 bursae scattered throughout our bodies. Although they are not part of the joint structure itself, bursae help us move by lubricating the areas near joints. The fluid produced by the bursae help muscles move more easily across muscles and over bones.

If exposed to prolonged stress or pressure, one or more bursae may become inflamed, and a condition known as bursitis develops. Sometimes bursitis also develops in people with arthritis because of an infection. The condition can come on very suddenly and catch you by surprise.

"Housewife's knee," or prepatellar bursitis, for instance, can develop if you kneel for prolonged periods on a hard surface; this might be the case if you cleaned a floor weekly. "Clergyman's knee," or tibial tubercle bursitis, can result if you kneel for prolonged periods on a more upright surface such as a kneeler in a church pew. "Student's elbow," or olecranon bursitis, can develop if you press your elbow against a desk or other hard surface for prolonged periods.

But bursitis most often affects the shoulder, resulting in an aching pain on the top of your shoulder and even more pain if you lift and rotate your arm backwards. Stiffness is especially evident in the morning but loosens up as the day goes on.

Bursitis in the shoulder may develop after an injury to the area such as during a contact sport or if something heavy falls on you. The condition may also develop if you strain or injure muscles in the area either through overuse or because you have exercised without warming up properly. Or it may develop as a complication of certain types of arthritis.

Whatever the cause and whatever type of bursitis you develop, the good news is that for the most part this condition generally will heal—often in several weeks—on its own. The first step is to take it easy until the most visible signs of inflammation subside. Resting the affected area will speed healing more than anything else you can do, but you may also find it helpful to protect the area in some way, either by wrapping the injured knee or elbow with an elastic bandage or using a splint.

Resting the area doesn't mean complete inactivity. Gently moving the affected joint a few times a day will help prevent it from becoming stiff. The idea is to avoid strain, not movement. Some good exercises to do at this time include swimming and walking.

If the area feels warm to the touch, try applying ice or a cold pack to reduce inflammation. If it is still painful when the area is cool to the touch, heat or a warm bath makes many people feel better.

Once the pain and inflammation have subsided, the best thing you can do is exercise. Concentrate on strengthening muscles in the particular area affected to increase their ability to withstand the stresses and strains of normal life. To avoid a recurrence, make sure you warm up and cool down properly. (For more information on how to exercise, see chapter 3.)

You should also try to take frequent short breaks while doing any type of repetitive task. Taking a five-minute break to stretch or even walk away from your desk will limber you up and provide the affected area with a needed rest.

For more advanced or persistent cases there are many over-the-counter NSAIDs such as aspirin and ibuprofen (brand names *Advil* and *Nuprin*) that provide extra pain relief. Applying ice to the area can also help.

If your bursitis fails to respond to these initial treatments, your healthcare provider may recommend an injection of a corticosteroid to reduce inflammation and refer you to a physical therapist.

Tendinitis

Dave was a weekend warrior. After a week in the office, he was ready to tackle the yard and breathe some air. But he must have overdone it this weekend. Somehow between cutting the lawn and clearing out all the brush at the back of the yard, he pulled something. His left elbow ached.

Tendons are tough, fibrous cords that connect muscles to bones at the joints. Tendinitis occurs when one or more tendons become inflamed. Sometimes the condition develops after an injury to a joint. At other times it develops because muscles are overworked or have become weakened. Both of these scenarios place more stress on the tendons, causing them to become inflamed.

Tendinitis results in anything from a dull ache to a sharp pain near the joint, and the area may become red and swollen. Sometimes movement is restricted; for example, you may not be able to raise your arm above a certain point. In fact, you may even think it is arthritis. But tendinitis affects the area just outside the joint, not inside it.

As in the case of bursitis, the best thing to do is rest the affected area until the pain and inflammation subside and try not to put any extra strain on the joint. If tendinitis resulted from exercising (after running, for instance), then take a few days off.

If the area is warm and swollen, apply ice or a cold pack to help stop the process of inflammation. If it still feels stiff and painful once the inflammation subsides, try heat to help the soft tissues heal.

Gently move the affected joint a few times a day to prevent stiffness. Swimming and walking would be good to do at this time.

To prevent recurrences of tendinitis, you may want to combine strength training (to build your muscles and take the strain off tendons) with flexibility exercises (which will lengthen the muscles and make the whole area less prone to injury). For more information about ways to exercise, see chapter 3.

For persistent cases of tendinitis you may want to try an over-the-counter NSAID such as naproxen sodium *(Aleve)* for extra relief.

If the problem persists, contact your healthcare provider. He or she may recommend ultrasound in which high-frequency sounds are directed at the affected tendon. This seems to speed healing and reduce inflammation.

Another option is to inject corticosteroids around the tendon to alleviate pain and inflammation, a strategy used most often in the shoulders and wrists. The achilles tendon should never be injected because of the risk of tendon rupture.

Repeated bouts with tendinitis may result in scar tissue on the tendons. In some cases your healthcare provider may recommend surgery, but this is generally regarded as a treatment of last resort and is not very effective.

Carpal Tunnel Syndrome

Diane was in charge of data processing at a law firm. She spent hours every day inputting data and preparing bills and reports. She knew she should take more breaks, but the pressure was intense and the workload never seemed to diminish. Lately she was wondering if she was working too hard. She noticed a tingling in her thumb and fingers, and sometimes her hand went numb. What was this?

Carpal tunnel syndrome affects the section of your arm between the forearm and wrist where the median nerve connects to your hand. This passageway, formed by bones on three sides and ligaments on the fourth, resembles a tunnel. Carpal tunnel syndrome develops when tendons near the bones that form the back side of the carpal tunnel become inflamed or when the ligament that forms the front side of the tunnel becomes thicker. As a result, the median nerve is compressed; this nerve supplies feeling to your thumb, index finger, long finger, and ring finger, and helps to move your thumb. When carpal tunnel syndrome develops and the nerve becomes compressed, the result is pain, numbness, and tingling in your fingers or even the entire hand, and pain in the wrist.

These symptoms may also indicate tendinitis or another disorder related to overuse of the joints, but even if you are not suffering from carpal tunnel syndrome, the advice that follows will help alleviate symptoms and prevent further problems.

The symptoms of carpal tunnel syndrome usually emerge slowly and progress gradually. At first you may notice mild pain and tingling when doing something that requires repetitive motions, but these symptoms may disappear when you stop. If the condition gets worse, you may notice that you drop things more often than you used to. The pain and tingling may intensify, may occur even when you are not using the affected arm, or may occur at night after going to bed. Or you may lose your ability to feel hot or cold objects.

About 3 million people have carpal tunnel syndrome each year. And as the population ages and as workplaces become more automated (resulting in more repetitive tasks), the incidence may increase. Fortunately, carpal tunnel syndrome can be prevented, and if you do develop the condition, it can be treated.

Since repetitive motions of the hands and wrists for prolonged periods of time, especially with extra pressure on the joints, may cause carpal tunnel syndrome, those in the meat- or fish-packing and construction industries are at highest risk, as are those who use a jackhammer for hours each day.

But office workers who use computers are also at risk, especially if they have poor posture; slouching while you type increases the risk. As you slouch, you bend your wrist, further compressing the nerve.

Some studies have shown that even psychological stress, either in the workplace or at home, can increase the chances of developing carpal tunnel syndrome (as well as other forms of musculoskeletal injury). This probably has to do with the fact that when we are feeling pressured, we tend to tense up, increasing the chance of injury.

Finally, carpal tunnel syndrome can also occur as a result of some other injury or illness, such as breaking an arm; the carpal tunnel may be damaged and place pressure on the nerves. The syndrome may also develop as a result of rheumatoid arthritis and other inflammatory conditions that can damage the tissues in the carpal tunnel.

Some people are more susceptible than others because of biological or hereditary factors. Some studies have also reported that it develops more often in women than in men. And some women have found that their symptoms worsen when they have premenstrual syndrome or are pregnant.

How to Protect Yourself

The Occupational Safety and Health Administration recently issued its first guidelines for ergonomics in the workplace. These guidelines are designed to protect you from the types of tasks and situations that might result in carpal tunnel syndrome and other types of musculoskeletal disorders. It will take employers some time to come up to speed about the new regulations. In the meantime, you can take a few commonsense and relatively simple steps to protect yourself.

If you have a job that requires you to do repetitive tasks for any extended period of time, try to take frequent short breaks to relieve the pressure on your hands. This can be as simple as taking your hands off the keyboard occasionally and shaking them or flexing the fingers, to keep everything limber.

If you work in an office, make sure that your chair is in a comfortable position that will enable you to work without strain. It should be high enough so that your elbows are bent at 90-degree angles and your hands reach the keyboard comfortably. Your wrists should be straight—not bent up or down at an angle. (Hang your arms by your side and notice how your wrists are straight.) Make sure the back of the chair is adjusted so that it provides your back with sufficient support. Try to sit up straight with your spine pushed against the back of the chair, chest jutting out slightly.

You might find it helpful to have a small pillow or support in the small of your back. You can also get a wrist support to place near the keyboard to force your wrists to remain straight at all times. If you can, adjust the tension on the keyboard so that it is easier to press the keys. In addition, many ergonomically designed office products are available that will further enable you to adapt your work environment.

If you work in construction or in a manufacturing plant, talk with your boss. You may not be able to do much about the equipment you have to use, but you can vary tasks so that you are not always using something like a jackhammer. Some tools, such as hammers and screwdrivers, are now being designed so that the pressure of holding and using them is distributed across the entire hand rather than centered in the palm. These may be worth investing in, or see if you can take short but frequent breaks from the assigned task.

Exercises

No matter what type of work you do, it's a good idea to strengthen the muscles in your hands and arms. This will better enable you to withstand the pressure of repetitive motion and reduce your chance of injury.

Start by warming up before you start to work. Flex your hands and fingers or rotate your shoulders a few times. The idea is to loosen up and try to keep limber throughout the day. You can do the following exercises at the work site or in an office. Try them a few minutes every hour and see if it helps make you feel better.

Hand exercises. Make a tight fist, then release and spread your fingers as far as possible. Repeat five times. Do the same with the other hand.

Holding your palm up, bend your thumb against the palm and hold for five seconds. With your thumb still bent, spread your fingers and hold for another five seconds. Repeat five to ten times, then do the same thing with the other hand.

Now concentrate on your wrists: Make a loose fist with your right hand, with the palm facing up. With your left hand, press down on the fist gently. Exert enough force to resist with your right hand, making sure that you keep your wrist straight. Hold for five seconds. Then turn the fist downward and repeat, pressing with your left hand against the knuckles on your right. Hold again for five seconds. Turn the right hand thumb side up, with the palm facing left. Take your left hand and press down gently on your right. Hold for five seconds. Reverse hands and repeat the sequence.

You can also flex the wrists by doing a simple stretch exercise. Hold your right hand up by your shoulder, palm facing outward, in a pose that may remind you of being a Boy Scout or Girl Scout taking a pledge. Take your left hand and bend your right hand backward gently, while the fingers remain together. Hold for five seconds. Finally, spread the fingers on your right hand apart while continuing to hold the pose for another five seconds. Repeat with the other hand.

Arm and shoulder exercises. Strengthening the muscles in your arms and shoulders can also reduce the risk of developing carpal tunnel syndrome. To stretch the muscles in your forearms, which can tighten up if you hold your hands in a particular position for a long time, do this exercise: Place your two palms together, fingers pointed up as if you were praying. Raise your elbows as far as you can until you feel a slight stretch in your forearms. Hold the position for ten seconds. Shake your arms a bit to loosen them and repeat.

To stretch the muscles in your neck and shoulders, place your right hand on top of your left shoulder while you are sitting down. Gently push the left shoulder down while turning your head to the right and looking down. You should feel a gentle stretch on the left side of your neck. Change hands and repeat with the right shoulder. Hold each position about five seconds.

You can also loosen your neck and shoulder muscles. Stand up with your arms dangling by your side. Roll your head forward, to the right, backward, and then to the left, stopping at each point for about five seconds. When you complete the circle, do an exercise with your shoulders: Shrug your shoulders up toward your ears, then back toward your spine, then down toward your feet, and finally forward. Pause a few seconds at each stop.

In addition to these exercises, which are specific to the upper portion of your body, you can protect yourself by developing an overall health and fitness plan. For more information on how to do so, see chapter 3.

Treatment Strategies

If you continue to have pain, tingling, and other symptoms of carpal tunnel syndrome that are not relieved by rest and simple exercises, try an over-the-counter pain reliever such as aspirin or ibuprofen (brand names *Advil* or *Nuprin*). If the pain persists, you may want to consult your healthcare provider about other options. He or she may suggest you wear a splint to keep your wrists straight. This will help inflammation subside and further protect the area against strain. You may also want to talk with your boss about workplace accommodations.

You should also ask for a referral to a physical and/or occupational therapist who can work with you to assess how you sit and hold your hands and arms—and how you might make some changes to your posture or work environment that will help you. He or she may also provide additional exercises and show you how to do them. See chapter 10 for more details.

If these initial strategies don't work, your healthcare provider may suggest that you start taking stronger NSAIDs to reduce pain and inflammation. (For more information see chapter 5.) If NSAIDs don't work, he or she may suggest corticosteroid injections or that you undergo ultrasound in which your wrist and arm are exposed to sound waves. Ultrasound seems to speed healing and relieve inflammation in some people. Surgery may also be an option if nothing works for you.

Complementary Therapies

You may want to supplement exercise and medication with complementary therapies that can make you feel better and may even help you heal. These include acupuncture (see chapter 11) and yoga (see chapter 12).

Surgery

In the most severe cases, where nothing else has worked, your healthcare provider may recommend surgery. The most common type for carpal tunnel syndrome is open release surgery in which the surgeon makes an incision in the palm and releases the ligament roof of the carpal tunnel, thereby decreasing the pressure on the median nerve. Or your surgeon may recommend a less invasive procedure that requires a smaller incision in the palm.

Recovery time and outcome depend on the type of surgery as well as age, overall health, and other medical conditions. Surgery rarely results in infections and other complications. Most people who undergo release surgery do find that they lose a fair amount of strength in their wrists for a few weeks, which is an important factor if you have a job that requires a lot of lifting (or if you have young children or grandchildren that you need to carry).

Many people have found that surgery solved the problem, but for some the pain persists or returns. If you are thinking about surgery, talk it over carefully with your healthcare provider and weigh the risks against the benefits.

Fibromyalgia

Nancy had her own painting business for several years and was happy to be making a good living without being stuck inside of an office. Then one day she woke up and felt as if she had the flu—sort of a dull ache all over. She took an over-the-counter medication, but the flu hung on and the ache increased. She went to her healthcare provider, but she could find nothing wrong. Nancy tried to ignore it, but the pain built slowly and steadily. A year later she could barely hold a paintbrush, it hurt so badly. And even the smell of the paint made her sick. She stopped working. After going to three healthcare providers, she found someone who could put a name to this misery.

Fibromyalgia is a stealth syndrome: It often eludes detection. If you have fibromyalgia, you may feel gnawing pain, a constant tiredness, and a depression so palpable it weighs on you. A healthcare provider may find nothing wrong. Blood tests may be normal and X rays look fine. The healthcare provider may think you have chronic fatigue syndrome because you are so exhausted, and you may begin to wonder if it is all in your head.

Fibromyalgia affects about 4 million people (women more often than men), making it twice as common as rheumatoid arthritis. Yet the condition remains poorly understood and hard to diagnose. All too often it is dismissed as a psychological problem. Fibromyalgia is a pain syndrome aggravated by tender points in the muscles that are much more sensitive to stimuli than other areas. It can occur on its own or in conjunction with other disorders such as an underactive thyroid condition.

Fortunately, in the past decade much has been learned about how to recognize and treat this syndrome. Although there is no cure for fibromyalgia, you do have options that will relieve pain and other symptoms.

Symptoms

In fibromyalgia the pain emanates from the area where the muscles, tendons, and ligaments attach to your bones. Areas most affected include the neck, knee, shoulder, elbow, and hip, but most people ache all over. The pain may be a general sore ache, or it may be sharp and burning or gnawing. It may ebb at certain times of the day, but it is always there.

Specific parts of your body may be especially tender and painful to the touch. You may also have trouble sleeping. You may fall asleep as soon as you go to bed but then wake up several times during the night. And no matter how much you sleep, you may still feel exhausted. You may suffer more headaches than usual, and when you do, the pain is more intense. You may be bloated. You might have constipation or diarrhea.

Because fibromyalgia amplifies sensations in many people, you may become sensitive to certain smells, lights, and noises.

You may also suffer intense bouts of anxiety or feel so depressed that you don't want to get out of bed in the morning. Or you may have trouble concentrating. You may experience numbness and tingling in your fingers and wonder if you have carpal tunnel syndrome.

Why Fibromyalgia Develops

Fibromyalgia tends to develop after some type of significant stress, such as an injury or illness. We still don't know what causes it, but studies conducted over the last decade or so have yielded intriguing clues and theories.

One theory is that the problem may begin when there is an imbalance in neurotransmitters, chemicals produced in the central nervous system that help the brain send and receive signals. Some studies have shown that people with fibromyalgia may produce too much substance P, which helps to send pain signals, and too little serotonin, which helps to block them. (Serotonin also is one of the neurotransmitters involved in regulation of mood and sleep.)

What You Can Do to Help Yourself

The first step in learning how to take charge of your fibromyalgia is to learn more about the condition. Your healthcare provider may have pamphlets, books, or videos that you can borrow. The Arthritis Foundation is an excellent source of information and produces brochures, newsletters, and a book about fibromyalgia. You may also ask your healthcare provider for a local support group.

The next step is to start exercising on a regular basis. That may seem like the last thing you want to do, especially if you're tired and your muscles ache, but the pain and fatigue will only worsen if you become sedentary because your muscles will start to weaken and your overall health will suffer.

Start slowly, with low-impact exercises such as walking and biking. Swimming is also an excellent way to get started; the water helps support your body weight so that you are not putting any extra strain on your joints.

It's also important to do flexibility exercises to stretch your muscles, which tend to become tighter with age and inactivity. The key is to start slowly and gradually increase the time you can hold the stretch. (See chapter 3 on the benefits of exercise and for some good examples of flexibility exercises.)

Finally, it's important to learn new ways to relax. Pain can make you tense up, and so can anxiety. Yoga and tai chi are two excellent ways to relax your body while also stretching muscles and improving flexibility (see chapter 12).

Medication Strategies

Because the main problem in fibromyalgia is pain, over-the-counter pain relievers provide relief for some people. These medications block pain signals in various ways and include such brands as *Tylenol* and *Bufferin*. (See chapter 5 for more information on how to treat pain.)

If simple pain relievers don't work, your healthcare provider may prescribe an antidepressant. This type of medication is effective in some people because fibromyalgia, like depression, may result from abnormally low levels of serotonin, a brain chemical that helps regulate moods but is also involved in muscle contractions. Some antidepressants inhibit the ability to absorb serotonin and thus enable more of it to circulate. Typical antidepressants used are amitriptyline (marketed under the brand name *Elavil*), cyclobenzaprine *(Flexeril)*, and fluoxetine *(Prozac)*.

If you do not respond to common pain relievers or antidepressants, your healthcare provider may recommend a stronger type of prescription pain reliever such as tramadol *(Ultram)*. Narcotics should be avoided in fibromyalgia syndrome because they can be addictive.

NSAIDs, which are used to treat many types of arthritis, may be used because of their pain-relieving effects rather than their ability to reduce inflammation. Corticosteroids have not been shown to be of much use in treating fibromyalgia.

Complementary Therapies

Because medication strategies do not work for everyone, you may also want to look into complementary approaches for managing your fibromyalgia. A brief description of the techniques believed useful in treating fibromyalgia follow. Much more detail is provided in chapter 11.

Acupuncture. Acupuncture gets mixed reviews, but it is helpful for some people with fibromyalgia. In this therapy needles are inserted into various parts of the body believed to be involved in the transmission of pain. (Sometimes tiny electrical jolts are given to interfere with the pain signals.) Some people with fibromyalgia find this helpful; others do not. The research continues.

Biofeedback. This approach is based on the theory that you can learn to control your perception of and reaction to pain. Therapists who use this technique attach some type of sensor to the part of your body that is bothering you. This sensor, which is painless, measures such things as your temperature, muscle contractions, and heart rate. The therapist will then work with you to find ways to relax. The sensors provide feedback based on their readings about whether the relaxation techniques are working (hence the name biofeedback). In time you will learn how to relax your muscles voluntarily without the sensors attached. How effective is biofeedback? Some people with fibromyalgia find it helpful; others do not. Clinical data is contradictory, and more research is needed.

Dietary supplements. Some people with fibromyalgia find that they feel better when they take a magnesium supplement. This mineral helps keep bones and other tissues healthy. It may be worth a try, but be sure to check with your healthcare provider first. Too much magnesium can be toxic, and it can interact with other medications, such as blood pressure medicine.

Magnets. It may seem strange to think that magnets could ease pain, but some people think they can. The theory is that magnets stimulate the electrical circuits in our bodies and improve circulation, encourage healing, and somehow interfere with the pain process. There have been few studies about this therapy, and the results are inconclusive.

Melatonin. This hormone has been touted for use in everything from sleep to sex disorders. Melatonin helps to regulate sleep and wakefulness. If you are having trouble sleeping or find that when you wake you feel exhausted, you may want to give this a try. But check with your healthcare provider first. Melatonin is not recommended if you are depressed (as many people with fibromyalgia are), and the studies about its use in fibromyalgia are inconclusive.

Relaxation techniques. Because you will feel better if you learn how to relax, you may want to investigate some popular relaxation techniques, such as massage, meditation, self-hypnosis, and yoga. Most are offered in your community.

What does not work. Some people think guaifenesin, which is found in many cough medicines, will cure fibromyalgia, but a study funded by the National Fibromyalgia Research Foundation showed no beneficial effect.

The Arthritis Connection

Question: How do I tell if my pain is a result of arthritis or another condition, such as bursitis and tendinitis?

Answer: Only your healthcare provider can tell for sure. It is difficult for a layperson to distinguish between the pain of arthritis and the pain of bursitis or tendinitis. If you have pain that frequently awakens you from sleep, it may be a sign that you have bursitis or tendinitis, not arthritis. Carpal tunnel syndrome is easier to distinguish, partly because of its distinct location in your lower arm and partly because it may result in numbness and tingling, which are not characteristic of most types of arthritis.

Question: If I have bursitis, tendinitis, or carpal tunnel syndrome, am I more likely to develop arthritis?

Answer: These conditions are better understood as "wake-up" calls to make you aware of your joints and the problems that can result if you don't take proper care of them. Once the initial symptoms have subsided, take time to protect your joints, build the muscles around them, and attend to your overall health. Having these conditions does not mean that you are at an increased risk for developing arthritis.

Questions to Ask Your Healthcare Provider

For bursitis, tendinitis, or carpal tunnel syndrome:

1. How can I adjust my daily activities to lessen the strain on my muscles and joints?
2. How long should I rest my joint before resuming my regular routine?

3. Are there any exercises you recommend?
4. Do you recommend medication?
5. How can I take steps to avoid developing arthritis?

For fibromyalgia:

1. How can I avoid triggering the pain?
2. Do you recommend any exercises or physical modalities?
3. Do you recommend any medications?
4. What are the side effects?
5. Where do I find a support group?

CHAPTER 10

The Essential Adjuncts—Physical and Occupational Therapy

Linda was shocked to hear that she had rheumatoid arthritis, and for a while she was depressed. "I'm too young," she thought, "and too healthy for this." But once the shock began to wear off, her resolve kicked in. "I got through natural childbirth fifteen years ago. No medication. Just learning how to breathe and work with my body instead of against it. If I could get through that, I can learn to manage this."

Frank was a football star in high school. He prided himself on playing even after he got hurt, and he got hurt a lot back then. He never thought about arthritis until the first real pain set in. His knees were the worst. Some days he could barely get off the bleachers after watching a baseball game. He wanted more than the medications his healthcare provider recommended. He wanted to keep moving. He wanted a new game plan.

Focus on Function

A diagnosis of arthritis can shake you emotionally. It changes your image of yourself and makes you feel old. Even if your symptoms are mild and your options many, arthritis is a word you don't want to hear with your name attached. It has too many negative connotations in our society: age, disability, limitation, loss.

It doesn't have to be that way. Physical and occupational therapy—and the philosophies that guide these professions—will help minimize your symptoms and ensure that you continue living your life pretty much as you did before you learned you had arthritis.

The goals of physical and occupational therapy are to decrease your pain, increase your mobility, and improve your balance and coordination. The focus is primarily on function—helping you retain your ability to do everyday tasks such as cooking and typing on a keyboard or helping you regain those abilities if they have been compromised by your arthritis.

There is a lot of overlap between the work of physical and occupational therapists. To distinguish between the two professions: *Physical therapists* focus on the entire body and tend to use exercises or adaptive devices to strengthen muscles. They also rely on heat, cold, braces, and splints to reduce pain and inflammation. *Occupational therapists* tend to focus on the upper extremities, especially the hands and arms. They also adapt equipment to make activities of daily living easier.

Ideally, you should see a physical or occupational therapist as soon as you are diagnosed with arthritis. Most often you will require only one or two visits before you are able to carry on at home or at work using the advice and exercises your therapist has provided.

If you are unable to visit a physical or occupational therapist early on, there are steps you can take to find relief and protect your joints.

Step 1: Stop the Pain and Inflammation

No matter what type of arthritis you have, chances are that at the beginning one or two joints will be especially painful. They may also be red, swollen, and warm to the touch—an outward sign of inflammation. Pain and inflammation can both interfere with your ability to move your joints and do things you never thought about before, including getting out of bed in the morning (you may feel stiff and stumble), getting up out of your chair, opening jars, and even buttoning clothes.

The first thing to do is focus on alleviating the pain and any inflammation. Then you can do specific exercises to regain function and range of motion.

To alleviate pain on your own, try applying heat or cold to the area. But how to figure out whether you should apply heat or cold? The easiest way to remember is this: If your skin feels warm to the touch, apply something cold. If your skin feels cool or the way it usually does, apply heat.

The reason has to do with blood flow. Heat tends to increase blood flow to the affected area. When your joint is warm and red, you already have increased blood flow to the area. If you apply something warm, you'll only prolong inflammation. Cold packs and ice will discourage blood flow and thereby alleviate inflammation. Once it has subsided, however, heat can alleviate pain and speed healing, partly by relaxing muscles. (Not all of the ways that heat works is understood, but it does work.)

Heat. You can apply heat to affected joints at home by taking a warm bath or shower, or by using a heating pad or a hot water bottle. Usually twenty to thirty minutes of heat application will be enough to relieve pain and relax muscles.

Another option is to try to capture and retain your own body heat. Joint warmers or certain support stockings keep joints warm while providing extra support. You might try wrapping yourself in blankets or layers of clothing for thirty minutes before exercising; you'll find that your muscles move more easily. Layering blankets on the bed or even using a sleeping bag at night may help with the stiffness you experience in the morning.

Still another option is to purchase a lotion or gel that warms the area where it is applied. Many of these are available at pharmacies, but check with your physical or occupational therapist first because some may not be appropriate for your type of arthritis.

Cold. The application of cold packs or ice to the affected area may also alleviate pain. Cold numbs the area, including nerves, so that pain seems less intense. It also decreases inflammation and reduces muscle spasms. Your physical or occupational therapist may recommend that you apply cold temporarily but not recommend it as a regular therapy. Prolonged exposure to cold may cause muscle stiffness, which will only exacerbate your symptoms.

To apply cold at home, try an ice pack. Ice cubes from your freezer will do nicely as long as they're placed in a plastic bag to prevent leaking and wrapped in a dish towel or something similar to make it more comfortable. Or you can buy an ice pack at your neighborhood pharmacy. Some stores sell gel packs that can be placed in the freezer and then applied. Or try applying a bag of frozen vegetables; it sounds strange, but it works. Another option is a topical lotion or spray to cool the area. These are also available at your local pharmacy.

Apply the cold pack to the affected joint for as long as it takes to feel better (and as long as you can stand it) but no longer than thirty minutes at a time.

Step 2: Protect Your Joints

You can prevent more pain and inflammation from developing by putting less pressure on your joints throughout the day. This will take some concentration at first because it involves relearning tasks that you barely think about—everything from opening jars to writing letters to walking. Some of our suggestions may seem trivial—does it really matter how you do your hand wash, for instance?—but if you revise the way you do many small tasks as you go through the day, by the time you go to sleep you will have saved your joints from pounds of cumulative pressure.

Before you can protect your joints, you first have to think about how you put them under pressure. The risk factors fall into three categories:

1. Position. Holding your body in an awkward way or twisting it into an unnatural position can increase the pressure placed on joints as well as on muscles and tendons. For instance, the right way to lift something is to keep your back straight while kneeling down to pick it up and then standing or by standing close to the object as you lift it. All too often we bend our backs to reach something and pick it up. Bending over places ten times the amount of pressure on our lower backs so that a 5-pound object places 50 pounds of force on our spines.

Likewise, our wrists are meant to be held straight (as they are when we dangle our arms). If you bend them as you type, you put more strain on the bones, muscles, and nerves in your hands and wrists.

2. Force. This factor puts more pressure on joints than is healthy. When you walk on concrete or pavement, you place more force on joints than if you walk on sand or grass, which have more natural "give" and therefore absorb some of the impact. Likewise, if you bang a hammer hard, your hands and elbow will feel the impact. Even writing with a pen and pencil can be hard on your hands. Think about how you hold the pen, especially if you are tense or on deadline. Are you gripping it tightly and bearing down hard on the paper? Are your hands and fingers sore afterward?

3. Repetition. Think about the activities you do again and again. If you work in an office, do you spend your whole day at a keyboard? Do you work on an assembly line doing the same thing over and over? On the weekend, do you try to trim all the bushes at once with a hedge clipper? Anytime you move your joint in the same way repeatedly you are placing cumulative stress on the joint—and that can lead to problems.

Fortunately, you can reduce the pressure on your joints by doing things differently, as follows:

BACK

- Sleep on a firm mattress to provide proper support at night.
- When you lift something, stand as close to the object as possible so that your back is straight, bend your knees, and push upward with your legs.

HANDS

- To reduce the pressure on your thumb and fingers, buy easy-grip pens and pencils (with enlarged or textured bodies) or wrap them in foam grippers.
- To reduce pressure on your fingers and palm, use a can opener or rubber gripper to open jars.
- When preparing food, pull backward with your knife to cut food rather than pushing forward. This reduces the pressure on your fingers.

KNEES

- Avoid wearing shoes with heels higher than 2 inches.
- Buy shoes with adequate support in the soles. If you need extra cushioning, buy padded insoles.

• Walk on grass or other soft surfaces and avoid walking on concrete whenever possible.

Step 3: Conserve Your Energy

In this frantic, fast-motion world, it is easy to get caught up in the frenzy. And what is the result? At the end of the day you're tired and wiped out.

The problem is that when you are tired, you are much less likely to think about protecting your joints or want to exercise—two key facets of keeping pain and inflammation at bay and making sure your arthritis doesn't get any worse. And certain types of arthritis— notably rheumatoid arthritis—will decrease your overall energy level and increase your fatigue.

The solution is to start consciously conserving your energy. This may also improve your mood because you will have more energy for leisure activities that make you happy.

Just as you can protect your joints from cumulative stress by revising the way you do things throughout the day, you can also save a lot of energy by trying the following five suggestions:

1. Stand and sit up straight. Good posture saves energy because it enables you to take advantage of the natural support your body provides while placing less strain on your joints. It will therefore take less energy to work and lift objects.

2. Take frequent short breaks. Resting periodically throughout the day, even if only for ten minutes, allows your body to recharge itself. A twenty-minute nap (in the office with your door closed or at home) may provide a better boost than a cup of coffee in the afternoon.

3. Pace yourself. If you want to weed your garden, do one section at a time and then take a break. All too often we go at things with gusto—mowing the whole lawn at once or cleaning the whole house in order to get it out of the way. It is better to break a big task into smaller components and spread it out over the day or week.

4. Alternate hard tasks with easy ones. If something is physically or mentally challenging, it can take a lot of energy. It is best to alternate a hard task with one that is easier. If you hate to write and your report is due at noon, then chances are the morning will be stressful, so spend the afternoon catching up on reading your emails and mail. If you spend Saturday morning cleaning the house, spend the afternoon taking a walk or just reading.

   5. Get organized. How much energy is misspent because it takes us ten steps to do what could have been done in five? Gather your clothes the night before so you're not rushing around the following morning trying to put an outfit together. Make a shopping list before you go to the store so that you're not wandering around trying to remember what you need—and then you don't have to go out again because you forgot something important.

Step 4: Start Moving

   One of the dangers of arthritis is that the original problem can snowball. You are in pain, so you stop moving. But because you stop moving, your muscles begin to weaken, your overall fitness decreases, and you end up stiffer and more sore than before.

   As discussed in chapter 2, we now understand that strong and flexible muscles provide primary support to the joints, with cartilage providing secondary shock absorption. As we age, muscles naturally tighten and weaken, which means they provide less support to the joints. That is why it is so important to begin exercising as soon as your initial pain and inflammation have subsided. The best way to start is with some simple range-of-motion exercises that help stretch the muscles and make you more flexible. See Flexibility Exercises on pages 225 to 231.

   Once you have warmed up by doing the flexibility exercises, you should focus on strengthening particular muscle groups. As discussed in chapter 3, you strengthen muscles by forcing them to push against something. The resistance builds muscle. You can strengthen muscles by pushing or pulling against an outside force (either a weight machine at a gym or a stretch fabric known as a theraband or theratube) or you can push against the weight of your own body. See pages 231 to 233 for examples of good strengthening exercises for various joints.

Flexibility Exercises

The following exercises will help loosen your joints and stretch your muscles, which will make you more flexible.

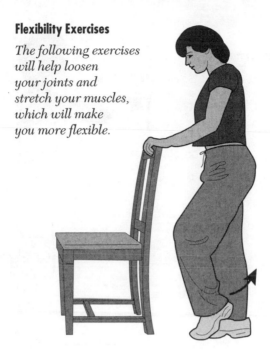

Ankles

1. Stand with your weight on your right leg, which should be slightly bent.
2. Hold on to a wall or a steady chair (not one with wheels) to support yourself.
3. Place your left heel on the floor while tilting your toes toward the ceiling.
4. Reverse so that the toes on your left foot touch the floor and your heel is raised.
5. Repeat 3 to 5 times.
6. Switch legs and repeat steps 1 through 5.

Knees

*Keep your movements
slow and fluid.*

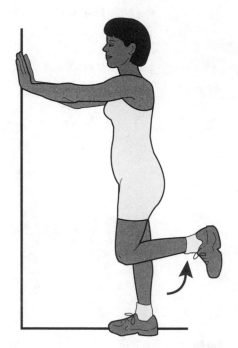

1. Stand with your hands on the back of a stationary chair or against a
   wall to support yourself.
2. Bend your leg and lift your right foot so that your heel points
   toward the ceiling.
3. Keep your back straight and your right thigh aligned with
   your left.
4. Lower your right foot.
5. Repeat steps 1 through 5 with the left leg.
6. Repeat 3 to 5 times for each leg.

Hips

If you need to support yourself during this exercise, stand to the side of a stationary chair, with your hand resting on its back.

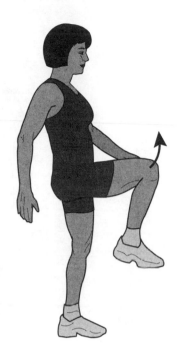

1. *Stand up straight.*
2. *Slowly lift your right foot off the ground in front of you as if you were marching in a parade.*
3. *Lift your knee so that it is at waist level and you can feel your hip joint move.*
4. *Lower your right foot.*
5. *Switch legs and repeat steps 1 through 4.*
6. *Repeat 3 to 5 times.*

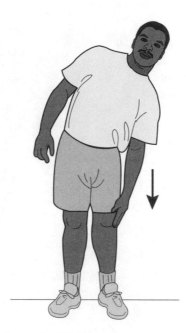

Lower Back

1. Stand with your knees slightly bent.
2. Place one hand on your abdomen and the other on your lower back.
3. Swing your hips forward so that your abdominal muscles tighten (you'll feel your spine curve outward).
4. Swing your hips backward so that your buttocks lift (you'll feel your spine tilt toward the front).
5. Repeat 3 to 5 times.

Middle and Upper Back

1. Stand up straight with your arms dangling by your sides.
2. Slowly slide your right hand down your right thigh, below your knee (or as far as you can reach). Keep your head and back straight as you do so. Don't lean forward or backward.
3. Return to standing position.
4. Slide your left hand down your left thigh, following the instructions above.
5. Repeat 3 to 5 times.

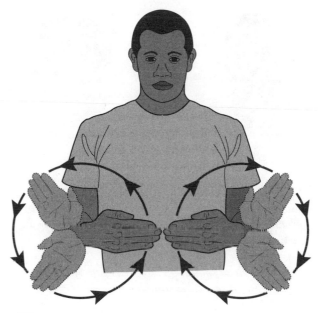

Hands and Wrists

1. Hold your arms close by your sides so that your elbows touch your waist.
2. Hold your hands in front of you so that they are at waist level (and your elbow is bent in a right angle).
3. Bend your hands inward so that your fingertips touch.
4. Make a circle with your hands so that your wrists bend up, in, down, and out.
5. Repeat the circles 3 to 5 times.
6. With your arms still tight against your body and your hands out in front of you, point your fingers outward toward the walls on either side of you.
7. Make circles in the air with your hands so that your wrists once again move up, forward, down, and in.
8. Repeat 3 to 5 times.

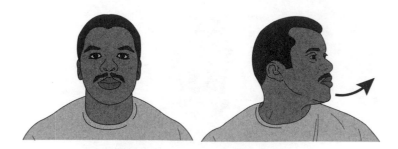

Neck

1. Stand and look in front of you.
2. Turn your head slowly to the right as if you were trying to look over your right shoulder. Keep your torso facing front; don't twist around. Only your head should move.
3. Hold the position for several seconds.
4. Slowly turn your head so that you look over your left shoulder.
5. Hold the position for several seconds.
6. Repeat 3 to 5 times.

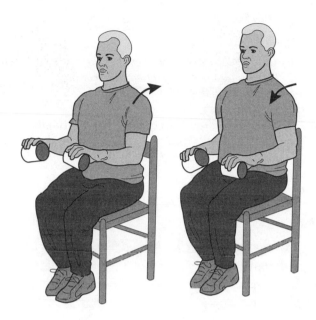

Shoulders

1. Sit in a stationary chair (not one with wheels).
2. Hold your arms close to your sides so that your elbows touch your waist and your hands are out in front of you.
3. Hold a weight in each hand with your palm facing downward. (You can buy hand weights in a store or use canned soups or vegetables from your cupboard.)
4. Push your shoulders back so that your chest thrusts outward and your elbows jut backward.
5. Hold the position for several seconds.
6. Relax your shoulders so that your elbows once again come forward toward your waist.
7. Repeat 3 to 5 times.

Strengthening Exercises

Shoulders

1. Stand up straight with your legs slightly apart for balance.
2. Lift your shoulders slowly toward the ceiling.
3. Drop them down toward the floor.
4. Repeat 3 to 5 times.
5. Pretend you are drawing a circle with your shoulders by lifting your shoulders up to the ceiling, curling your shoulders forward, dropping your shoulders down, and pushing your shoulders backward.
6. Repeat 3 to 5 times.

Thighs

This exercise is particularly good for your knees because it strengthens the muscles in your thighs.

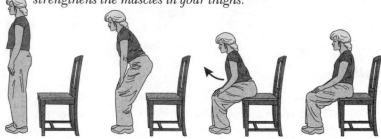

1. Sit in a stationary chair.
2. Lean forward slowly and stand by pushing up with your thigh muscles.
3. Stand up.
4. Slowly sit down by bending your knees so that your thighs do most of the work.
5. Repeat 3 to 5 times.

Alternate Exercise: Knee Bends

1. Stand with your legs apart and slightly bent.
2. Slowly lower your buttocks so that your knees bend and you feel your thigh muscles work. Move as if you were going to squat down but don't lower yourself that much!
3. Straighten up slowly.
4. Repeat 3 to 5 times.

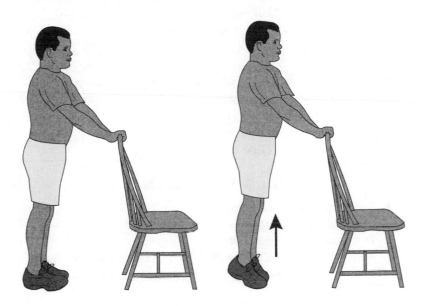

Calves

This exercise uses your own weight to provide resistance and build muscle.

1. *Stand up straight with your knees slightly bent.*
2. *Hold on to a wall or stationary chair for support.*
3. *Raise both heels off the ground.*
4. *Gradually lower them back down.*
5. *Repeat the up-and-down motion slowly until you become tired.*
6. *Shake your legs to loosen the muscles.*

The key to strengthening muscles is to repeat the motion ten to twelve times in a row without taking a break. You'll notice as you repeat the motion that it becomes increasingly hard to do. That's all right. The repetition helps build muscle as much as the resistance you are using.

As you exercise, listen to your body. If it hurts, stop immediately. You need to respect the pain of your arthritis: If it hurts, your joint needs more time to recover.

Exercise Do's and Don'ts

1. Start off slowly. Don't overdo it. Build slowly.
2. Always warm up and cool down.
3. Wear comfortable, loose-fitting clothes.
4. Apply heat or cold before you exercise if you are concerned about pain. Some people like to exercise right after a warm shower because their muscles feel looser.
5. Stop immediately if any of the following occur:

   - You have sharp pain in your joint or muscles.
   - You feel dizzy.
   - You feel nauseous.
   - You become short of breath. (It's okay to breathe harder but not to become severely breathless.)

Remember: One of the biggest mistakes people make is trying to "work through the pain." It's all right to feel sore after exercising, but if the pain is sharp or if it persists for more than an hour or so, you've overdone it.

Dealing with Common Problems

As we age we all tend to develop the same types of problems. Our backs begin to ache, we find it harder to crouch, or we can't grip a tennis racket as firmly as we did years ago. Some of this has to do with the fact that we lose strength and flexibility as we get older (see chapter 3). This may also be a sign that we are at risk of developing (or have already developed) arthritis.

What can you do? A few targeted exercises will help you deal with these common problems.

Backache

Lower back pain is one of the most common ailments of those middle aged and older. The pain may result from poor posture, which places undue strain on the vertebrae, or you may need to strengthen and stretch the muscles in your back.

Lower back. To gain flexibility in your lower back, try the "scary cat" stretch:

1. Get down on all fours on the floor.
2. Tuck your head and buttocks in as you arch your back (like a scary cat).
3. Slowly release the tension and raise your chin and buttocks toward the ceiling, so that you arch your back in a gentle U shape.
4. Repeat 5 to 10 times. You should feel more relaxed afterward.

Middle and upper back. You can also stretch the muscles in your middle and upper back, which in turn will help you move your shoulders and arms. See page 236.

Back Exercises

1. Stand with your legs slightly apart and your knees bent.
2. Thrust your hips slightly forward so that your abdominal muscles tighten.
3. Cross your arms in front of you.
4. Turn your whole torso to the right as you look over your right shoulder.
5. Slowly turn the other way so that you are looking over your left shoulder and your torso faces left.
6. Repeat 3 to 5 times.

This exercise is similar to the previous one, but you can sit down when you do it.

1. Sit in a stationary chair, looking straight ahead of you.
2. Turn your torso to the right so that you look over your right shoulder.
3. Turn until you can place your right arm on the back of the chair.
4. Place your left palm on your right knee and turn further.
5. Hold for several seconds.
6. Relax and return to the original position, facing straight ahead.
7. Repeat steps 1 through 5, but in the opposite direction.
8. Repeat 3 to 5 times.

Hand Weakness

Are you having a harder time opening jars? Do you fumble with your buttons as you get dressed? Have you been dropping things lately? These may all be signs that your hand muscles have become weaker and that you may have arthritis. Hand weakness is to some degree a function of age, but it can be reversed. Pay particular attention to the joint at the base of the thumb, in the fleshy part of your hand near your wrist. This is the basal joint. Many women and some men in their late forties and early fifties develop arthritis in this joint as a result of prolonged wear and tear.

You can improve your grip and regain your ability to perform everyday tasks by doing hand-strengthening exercises. To provide resistance, work with a ball of putty (available where toys are sold) or fill a sock with rice. The idea is to create a round object that has some "give" when you squeeze against it. See below for examples of how to strengthen your hands.

Hand-strengthening Exercises
Grasp

1. Place a ball of putty in the palm of your hand.
2. Squeeze gently so that you make a fist around the putty.
3. Squeeze a little harder.
4. Release.
5. Repeat 10 times, 3 to 5 times a day.

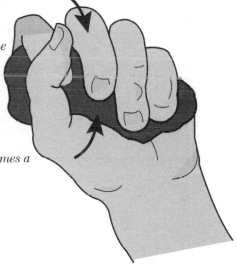

Fingertips

1. *Pinch putty between your thumb and index and middle fingers.*
2. *Squeeze gently and then harder, as if trying to touch your thumb with your fingers.*
3. *Relax.*
4. *Repeat 10 times, 3 to 5 times a day.*

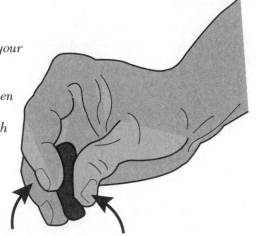

Side Pinch

1. *With hands held thumb side up, hold putty between your thumb and the upper side of your index finger.*
2. *Squeeze gently and then a little harder as if trying to touch your thumb and finger.*
3. *Release.*
4. *Repeat 10 times, 3 to 5 times a day.*

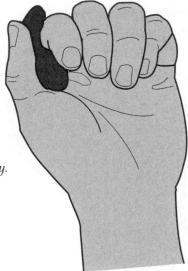

Finger Spread

1. *Place a small rubber band around your index and middle fingers.*
2. *Spread your fingers apart so that the elastic stretches.*
3. *Hold for 5 seconds.*
4. *Relax.*
5. *Repeat 10 times.*
6. *Now place the elastic around your ring finger and pinkie.*
7. *Spread the fingers apart so that the elastic stretches.*
8. *Hold for 5 seconds.*
9. *Repeat 10 times.*
10. *Do the entire sequence 3 to 5 times a day.*

Knee Aches and Pains

If your knees ache after a long walk, it could be a sign that your muscles are not providing enough support. (It could also mean that you need more support than your shoes are providing. See chapter 12 for what to look for in a shoe.)

You can ease the pain in your knees and minimize the symptoms of arthritis by strengthening the muscles that support your knees. Of particular importance are your quadriceps, the muscles in the front of the thigh. To strengthen your quadriceps, make it push repeatedly against some force—provided by a theraband or by your own weight.

Here's an exercise you can do in your office if you have a rolling chair:

1. Sit in the chair with your feet flat on the ground and your arms comfortably on the armrests or the side of the chair.
2. Push against the floor with your feet so that the chair rolls backward.
3. Repeat 5 to 10 times.

If you don't have much space in your office, you can roll in place by pushing off with your feet and then grabbing the desk with your hands to roll back into position.

See page 241 for some other good knee exercises.

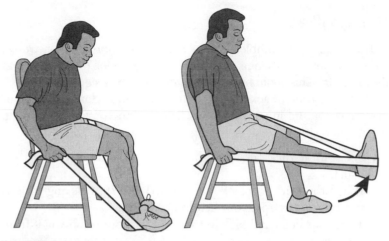

Knee Exercise

You can do the following exercise using ankle weights or a theraband tube. Or you can use tights or support stockings instead of a tube to provide some tension.

1. *Sit in a stationary chair with your feet flat on the ground.*
2. *Rest your palms on the side of the chair for support.*
3. *If you are using a stretch tube or theraband, loop it once around your right foot.*
4. *Slowly lift your right foot so that your leg straightens. You should feel your thigh muscle work as you lift the ankle weight or push against the theraband tube.*
5. *Hold your leg out straight for several seconds.*
6. *Slowly lower your foot to the ground.*
7. *Switch legs and repeat steps 1 through 6.*
8. *Continue until your legs feel tired.*

Morning Stiffness

Have you ever stumbled out of bed in the morning—or, worse, fallen? Sometimes it seems as if our feet and legs don't work as well as they used to. This could be a sign of age or an early sign of arthritis.

It may be time to acknowledge that you can no longer jump out of bed as you did in your twenties. If you find yourself stumbling, try the following to see if they help:

1. Set your alarm clock a half-hour or even an hour earlier than usual.
2. When the alarm goes off, stay in bed and start flexing various muscle groups from your head to your toes.
3. Turn your head and look to the right without removing it from the pillow.
4. Now look left. Repeat 5 to 10 times.
5. Stretch your arms up into the air or over your head as you do when you yawn. (And you may well be yawning in the morning.) Hold the stretch for several seconds, then relax. Repeat 3 to 5 times.
6. Flex your wrists by bending them back and forth and from side to side. Repeat several times in all directions.
7. Make a fist with both hands and then relax. Repeat 3 to 5 times.
8. Bring your right knee up to your chest. Hold for several seconds, then straighten your leg. Do the same with your left knee. Repeat 3 to 5 times.
9. To loosen your hips, keep your knees bent and tilt your legs first to the right, then to the left. Keep your knees together so that you rock back and forth, but keep your back flat on the mattress. Repeat 3 to 5 times.
10. Let your knees fall to either side so that you feel a gentle pull in your thighs. Hold the position for 15 to 20 seconds to stretch your thigh muscles.
11. Straighten your legs and flex your feet up and down at the ankles. Repeat 3 to 5 times.
12. Pull the covers back and sit up slowly. Let your feet dangle a minute or so before you try to stand.

Office Aches and Pains

Do you ache when you get up from your chair at the end of a business day? Do you sometimes feel stiff when you walk down the hallway? These may be signs that your body, and especially your joints, are under strain.

Although ergonomic devices are plentiful and can provide relief, your first step should be to reevaluate your own work habits. Do you sit up straight or do you slouch? Do you take regular breaks from your work or do you toil nonstop? To avoid aches and pains and to minimize symptoms if you have arthritis, try the following:

1. Sit up straight and use good body mechanics when working on a computer. Follow the guidelines in chapter 8.
2. When you retrieve a file, turn your whole body toward the file drawer. As you pull the drawer out with your right hand, brace yourself by placing your left hand on your left knee. (If you are left-handed, use the opposite hands.) This helps straighten your back and makes the task easier.
3. Don't twist part of your body. This only places more strain on whatever joints you are using. If you have to turn to accomplish a task, turn your whole body.
4. If you have to lift something, get as close to the load as possible. Bend your knees and tighten your abdominal muscles so that the load is placed on your lower extremities rather than on your back, hands, or arms.
5. Take breaks. Even if you don't leave your desk, you can do simple leg and ankle flexes to keep your muscles limber. Or take a walk down the hall just to get up and move. Stand up once in a while and arch your back, stretching your arms up in the air.

Know When to Seek Help

As much as you can try to help yourself, there are times when you should seek help from a physical or occupational therapist. How to know when to turn for help?

- You try the self-help steps included earlier in this chapter but still have difficulty with everyday tasks.
- You are in pain in spite of trying the steps outlined earlier.
- Your healthcare provider or rheumatologist recommends that you see a physical or occupational therapist.

The easiest way to find a physical or occupational therapist is to ask your healthcare provider or rheumatologist for a referral. It is likely that he or she regularly works with an individual or a group of therapists who can provide you with advice and instruction.

Also check with your health insurance plan. Some provide lists of preferred or authorized physical and occupational therapists. Some health plans also require that a referral be made by your healthcare provider or rheumatologist before they will pay for physical or occupational therapy charges.

Components of Your Therapy

Although the exact mix of modalities will depend on the type of arthritis you have and how severe it is, some of the following will probably be part of your therapy.

Diet. It's important to pay even more attention to proper nutrition once you have been diagnosed with arthritis. First of all, your body needs a regular supply of vitamins, minerals, and other nutrients to function well even under the best of circumstances. Now that you are living with a chronic disease, it's even more important to make sure that your body has all the energy it needs. Another issue to consider is that every extra pound you carry puts more weight on your joints, which are now less able to withstand that extra pressure. So it's good to start paying more attention to what you're eating during the day. Stay away from foods that are high in fat and low in nutrients; they add pounds without giving you much energy in return. For more information about the components of a healthy diet see chapters 3 and 12.

Pain relief. If the pain relief methods described earlier have not worked, your physical or occupational therapist may recommend other modalities such as:

TENS. Transcutaneous electrical nerve stimulation applies tiny electric currents to the areas that are painful. (This sounds worse than it is; the technique is not painful.) Typically, you would have a portable battery pack with electrodes that can be applied to your skin. You will be able to control when and where the currents are applied. Chances are you will not feel a shock or any type of pain; it will be more of a tickle or vibration. But TENS works by distracting your brain with these impulses so that it does not perceive—and you do not feel—the pain signals coming from the same area.

Ultrasound and other heat treatments. If your pain is severe or persists, the affected joint and surrounding tissue can be exposed to sound waves that penetrate deep into the body to warm the area.

Other heat treatments include infrared lamps, a special type of light that penetrates deep into tissues, or a heated whirlpool, or warm paraffin wax applied to specific joints.

Exercise. If you are seeing a physical or occupational therapist, chances are your joints hurt sufficiently that you will not be able to do some of the exercises mentioned earlier. Yet it is important to exercise, so that your muscles don't weaken and the original problem doesn't become worse.

Your physical or occupational therapist may suggest passive range-of-motion exercises. He or she will grasp your joint gently and move it slowly through its full range of motion. Or you can do the same thing. (For instance, if your shoulder is affected, take your upper arm and gently move it up, backward, down, and then to the front so that your shoulder moves.)

Your physical or occupational therapist may also suggest that you do isometric exercises in which you contract your muscles without actually moving your joints. This enables you to build muscles supporting the joint without putting any pressure on it. (See chapter 6 for an example of an isometric and an isotonic exercise.)

Assistive devices. These may include canes, splints, and walkers. Splints come in several varieties, for use on wrists, arms, and elbows. Braces are available for knees.

All these devices help you to rest your joint by taking some of the load off—literally. If your hands are sore after a day of keyboarding or if your arms ache after mowing the lawn, a splint may help. It wraps around the joint and provides support that muscles and tendons would normally provide while you accomplish the task.

Canes provide enormous relief to the lower extremities. When you walk with a cane, you hold it in the hand opposite your aching knee or ankle. This helps reduce the strain on your aching joint by half.

Some splints and braces can be purchased at the local pharmacy or through a medical supply store or catalog. Generally speaking, the more flexible the materials, the less support they provide to a joint. If you have mild to moderate pain when you use a joint, a splint made of cloth and leather may be enough. For more advanced problems, you may require one made of hard plastic.

These devices are often used temporarily and can be discarded once the joints have become stronger or healed. Ask your physical or occupational therapist how to camouflage splints and other devices if you are concerned about appearance.

Orthotic devices. Another way to provide support to joints, especially those in the ankles, feet, and knees, is to purchase orthotic devices for your shoes. Some orthotic devices provide better support and stabilize a particular part of the body, while others help to maintain balance; these include heel supports and sole inserts.

What Will Happen During Your First Visit

When you visit a physical or occupational therapist for the first time, he or she will assess your overall musculoskeletal health and functional abilities and then make recommendations about improving both. The first visit usually takes an hour.

Medical history. The visit may begin, as it did at your healthcare provider's office, with a medical history. Although your physical or occupational therapist should have your medical records, he or she may want to ask additional questions, including: What activities have been limited by your arthritis or its symptoms? What do you want to do either at work or at home that you can't do now?

What don't you want to give up? Do you have a spouse or significant other who can provide support? Do you know about support groups in your area?

Evaluation of musculoskeletal health. The next step is generally an assessment of your overall musculoskeletal health. Your physical or occupational therapist will actually measure your strength, range of motion, and functional ability. These will provide baseline measurements that will help shape your treatment plan. The therapist will look at both your active range of motion (how much you can move the joint on your own) and passive range of motion (how much he or she can move it while probing the area for signs of joint damage).

While making this evaluation, the therapist will probably ask you whether you have stiffness in any joints and, if so, when. This will help him or her to pinpoint specific muscles that need to be strengthened.

Strength. The physical or occupational therapist may also evaluate the strength of major muscle groups such as those in the shoulders, arms, back, and legs. This assessment may involve something as simple as pushing against the therapist's hand, to gauge your strength, or answering questions about the types of activities you do. The therapist may also have various electronic devices that can measure your muscle strength as you go through a series of resistance exercises.

Pain assessment. While evaluating your range of motion and strength, the physical or occupational therapist will also ask about the amount of pain you are experiencing as particular joints are moved. He or she may also provide some type of pain scale, usually a chart or graph, where you can indicate how much it hurts.

Don't worry that you will be forced to endure pain, though. Your physical or occupational therapist has not studied medieval torture. He or she will ask you to move your joints as much as you can but will not force you to hold a position that is painful. The evaluation determines at what point pain kicks in and, if it does, how much it hurts.

Assessment of functional ability. Your physical or occupational therapist may also ask you to stand up straight, walk across the room, sit down on a chair, and get up. He or she may ask how you get around town (walk? drive? take a bus?). Do you cook? Wash clothes? Garden? Mow the lawn? What do you do for a living? And with each set of questions, the therapist may ask you to demonstrate how you accomplish each task, and may even have sample tools or equipment so you can demonstrate.

This assessment will make you think about tasks you've probably given little thought to before. That is precisely the point. We don't realize how often we use our joints until they start to hurt. The therapist asks the questions in order to determine which tasks need to be rethought so you can perform them in a way that is less painful or less stressful to your joints.

Additional assessments. Depending on the type or severity of your arthritis, the therapist may also examine your skin for signs of disease or complication, and test your neurological responses to determine if there is any nerve damage.

Education and Instruction

After assessing your overall musculoskeletal health, your occupational or physical therapist will show you how to improve your posture while standing or sitting, how to take advantage of the support your spine can provide the rest of your body, and how to reduce the pressure you are inadvertently placing on your joints. He or she will also show you how to do simple exercises to strengthen and stretch certain muscle groups, and tell you how to improve your overall cardiovascular health by doing aerobic exercises.

Because it will take a while to learn how to do these exercises properly, your physical or occupational therapist will probably give you written instructions with diagrams to take home and practice. He or she may also provide books, pamphlets, and videos or tell you where to find them. If you need assistive devices, the therapist will probably be able to suggest where they can be purchased locally.

What Will Happen on Subsequent Visits

You might return to your physical or occupational therapist for a follow-up visit, either right after the first visit or some time later. Such follow-up visits can be helpful if you encounter difficulty with a particular activity and want advice about how to remedy it or if your arthritis should worsen. Or you might decide that you would like to see your therapist every year or so to make sure you are on track with your flexibility and strength exercises and other strategies for maintaining your mobility.

Typically, subsequent visits take much less time than the first, perhaps a half-hour instead of an hour. Your therapist has the records of your first visit and does not have to do a complete reassessment of your functional ability (although he or she may want to see how certain joints are doing).

Communicating with Your Healthcare Team

A brief word about communication: It is a good idea to make sure that your healthcare provider and your physical or occupational therapist are kept up to date about what the other is advising and doing. Ideally, these medical professionals will talk to one another about your situation or, at the very least, share office notes and medical charts. But sometimes things happen that prevent this, so it's best to keep the members of your healthcare team informed and in the loop.

You do not have to become a medical professional yourself; you just have to keep track of the various pieces of paper you'll be given and share them with each healthcare team member. Keep a file and place in it your symptom tracking chart, list of medications, exercise handouts, and any notes you may have taken during visits. After a visit to your physical or occupational therapist, ask how he or she will convey the assessment and therapy plan to your healthcare provider.

Questions for Your Physical or Occupational Therapist

1. How should I rest my joint so that my pain and inflammation will subside?
2. I'll know when the pain is gone, but how do I know when the inflammation is gone as well?
3. What type of exercises do you recommend?
4. What type of exercises should I avoid?
5. Where can I buy products that will make my life easier?
6. How do I adapt my work space to minimize the strain on my joints?
7. How can I do things differently at home to reduce the pressure on my joints?
8. How do I know if I've overused a joint?
9. How can I tell the difference between normal soreness and the type of pain that is a warning signal that I've overdone it?
10. Can you recommend any exercise books or videos suitable for me?

Likewise, on the next visit to your healthcare provider, mention your physical or occupational therapy program and how it's going.

However you accomplish it, remember that maintaining good communication between the members of your healthcare team will ultimately benefit you—and that's the whole point.

CHAPTER 11

Complementary Therapies

When Betty was diagnosed with rheumatoid arthritis two years ago, she felt betrayed by her body. Only thirty-eight at the time, she was otherwise fit and healthy. She had taken care of herself, watched her diet, exercised regularly—and then the diagnosis. The fact that her healthcare provider assured her that this type of arthritis could come out of nowhere and could affect anyone was of small comfort. Once she got over the shock, Betty carefully considered all her options. She took medications to control the inflammation and pain, visited a physical therapist early on to learn new exercises to maintain her muscle strength, and took a self-help course sponsored by the local chapter of the Arthritis Foundation. And last but in no way least, she began experimenting with different complementary therapies— everything from aromatherapy to yoga. Gradually she found a mix of therapies that supplemented her medical treatments and, for the first time in two years, made her feel as though she were back in control of her body instead of the other way around.

CHANCES ARE you have already tried some type of complementary therapy. If you have, you are in good company. One 1997 study estimated that four out of every ten Americans (and one out of every two who were thirty-five to forty-nine years old) had used at least one complementary therapy in the previous year, ranging from acupuncture to spiritual healing. About one in four people with arthritis said they had used some type of complementary therapy. (Other studies have estimated the number to be even higher.)

But just what is complementary therapy (also known as alternative medicine)? This broad term encompasses everything from acupuncture and bee venom to yoga and zinc supplements. By some estimates there are more than 130 complementary therapies; in addition, there are more than 500 unconventional remedies, including vitamin and other dietary supplements, herbs, and plant extracts.

Let us explore some of the major complementary therapies that have been popular with people who suffer from arthritis. We intentionally use the term "complementary" because we believe these therapies should supplement rather than replace more conventional therapies.

Herbs, Health, and Hype

Complementary therapies have increased in popularity over the past ten years. Most dramatic of all has been the use of herbal remedies, which grew 380 percent between 1990 and 1997, according to a study by David M. Eisenberg, M.D., and others. You may think that complementary therapies have just burst onto the scene, but in fact just the opposite is true. Many complementary therapies are based on ancient healing systems that predate the modern system of medicine that began in the twentieth century. Acupuncture, for instance, was first practiced thousands of years ago. And while taking herbal supplements may seem New Age, actually most of the medicines available before the arrival of chemistry and pharmacology were derived from common plants. So in some respects complementary therapy is a return to the past.

It is precisely this sense of "going back to the future" that divides proponents and opponents of complementary therapies. People who favor alternative approaches see them as providing a welcome relief from our modern medical system, which can seem cold and mechanized. Herbal supplements are also perceived as being gentler on the body than the arsenal of arthritis medications your healthcare provider may recommend. And if you have tried herbs and other complementary therapies and found them helpful, you may be convinced that they have improved your health.

But opponents of complementary therapies point out that modern medicine, for all its failings, has helped extend the average life span by almost thirty years—from forty-eight years at the turn of the twentieth century to seventy-six years at the beginning of the twenty-first. And they grumble that herbs and other dietary supplements are not regulated by any government agency, that they are not held to the same standards as pharmaceuticals. Complementary therapy, the critics say, provides more hype than hope.

We will walk on a middle path between the advocates and the critics of complementary therapy and explore the pros and cons of various alternative approaches. That way you can consider the information and make up your own mind.

Beware of "Cures" Touted in Glossy Advertisements

You may occasionally see glossy, full-color promotional materials that tout the latest arthritis "cure" or "breakthrough." Sometimes one substance is promoted; at other times a product that combines different ingredients is highlighted. These promotions may look professional and cite "scientific" evidence.

Listed below are some complementary therapies that are being advertised aggressively and why we think you should be skeptical of the claims they make:

- **Bromelain:** This substance, derived from pineapples, is touted as an anti-inflammatory agent. There is no valid scientific evidence that this is so.
- **CMO:** One study using mice found some value in this chemical, but it's a long jump from mice to men. Worse, people taking CMO for rheumatoid arthritis are advised to stop taking drugs like methotrexate, which has been shown to be of value.
- **DMSO:** This chemical, found in paint thinner, has been studied for use in treating arthritis. The research has been mixed, and we are not convinced it is safe. Our main concern is that you can't trust the DMSO you purchase commercially; the substance is seldom pure.
- **MSM:** This derivative of DMSO is being promoted heavily as a cure for a number of ailments. No studies of this substance have been done on people, and the fact that it is derived from DMSO worries us: It could contain the same impurities.

Why Complementary Therapies May Help

There are as many reasons that a complementary therapy may help you as there are different types. And it may surprise you to realize how close some of them are to mainstream medical advice. Complementary therapies that emphasize movement, such as tai chi and yoga, help build and maintain your muscles and overall physical fitness.

Those that encourage you to improve your "mind-body connection" or to relax can have significant impact on your perception of pain. Some reduce pain in measurable ways, as shown through clinical studies; these include acupuncture, biofeedback, and regular exercise.

But the jury is still out on other therapies that have shown early promise but need additional assessment before they can be recommended without reservation.

Although the news is mixed, we have devoted a chapter to this topic because the area shows much promise. And regardless of the exact mechanisms or effectiveness of individual therapies, complementary therapy provides what you need as you learn to live with your arthritis: a sense of control over your own body. By evaluating, choosing, and then integrating complementary therapies into your overall treatment regimen, you will be taking a more active role in the management of your disease. And that is invaluable.

Why Complementary Therapies Could Hurt

It may seem ridiculous that taking vitamins or herbal supplements could hurt you, but the truth is they could—under certain circumstances. In fact, some herbal remedies have been associated with abnormalities in heart rhythm, allergic reactions, high blood pressure, kidney and liver problems, and mania.

In excess amounts some herbs and supplements can interact adversely with other medications you are taking. And at high doses both vitamins A and D can be toxic.

With about one in five people on prescription medicines also taking a high-dose vitamin or herbal supplement, some experts estimate that about 15 million people are putting themselves at risk for an adverse interaction. Some pharmacies have begun to monitor for potential interactions between supplements and prescription medications; check to see if yours does and how you can take advantage of the service.

These remedies may also hurt your wallet. For the most part, alternative remedies don't come cheap. Some people begin taking a dietary supplement but then have to discontinue it because of cost. In fact, the Eisenberg team estimated that in 1997 people spent $27 billion out of their own pockets on complementary therapies—about the same as what they spent for physician services. See Table 14 for costs of sample therapies.

TABLE 14. Costs of Complementary Therapies

You may pay more—or less—depending on how much you buy at a time, where you live, and what brand you buy. Prices are based on the recommended doses for each product.

Because herbs and other dietary supplements are not drugs, they are generally not covered by health insurance plans.

Complementary Therapy	Sample Cost
Aloe gel	$3.50 to $10 per product
Boron	$1.40 to $2.90/month
Boswellia	$12/month
Chondroitin sulfate	$23 to $30/month
Evening primrose oil	$7.70 to $9/month
Fish oil (EPA)	$9 to $17/month
Flaxseed powder	$7 to $9 per 16 oz container
Glucosamine/chondroitin sulfate	$25 to $28/month
Glucosamine	$17 to $26/month
Kava supplements	$5.35 to $9/month
SAM-e	$79 to $210/month depending on brand and dose

Another significant risk is that of the unknown because dietary supplements are not regulated by the federal government.

Unregulated "Medicines"

As much as herbal remedies, vitamins, and dietary supplements may seem natural and therefore safe, the fact is that they are commercial products not regulated by the federal government. This is the result of the Dietary Supplement Health and Education Act of 1994, which created a new class of substances known as dietary supplements that are not considered drugs. Botanicals, herbs, vitamins, and nutritional supplements are all considered dietary supplements.

Dietary supplements do not have to go through clinical trials to meet standards of safety and effectiveness, and the FDA, which monitors the safety of the nation's food and drug supply, does not approve dietary supplements prior to sale. That means any claims made on the packaging or in advertisements should be considered marketing hype rather than medical advice. And many products are marketed aggressively without any real evidence to back up the claims.

Even when the remedy is helpful, there is no way of knowing whether a particular product contains the amount or type of ingredients listed on the container. There is also no assurance that the product is free of contaminants such as heavy metals or toxins. One analysis, of St. John's wort, found that only one brand contained the amount of active ingredient listed on the box (.3 percent of hypericin); four other brands contained amounts ranging from .25 percent to .28 percent. And glucosamine/chondroitin sulfate supplements, which have become increasingly popular as a complementary therapy for osteoarthritis, vary widely in amounts of active ingredients. In fact, some physicians recommend that you try another brand if you don't get any benefit from a particular glucosamine/chondroitin supplement within a month.

Anecdote Versus Evidence

Because herbs and other dietary supplements are exempt from FDA review, there has been little motivation for manufacturers to submit them for objective study, and only recently have mainstream researchers in the United States begun to conduct clinical studies. The impetus has come from the National Center for Complementary and Alternative Medicine, a division of the National Institutes of Health. But so far not much published data have resulted. Some complementary approaches have been studied in other countries, but the studies have been challenged for faulty design or for using standards different from those used in the United States.

In the absence of objective evidence, what we have to go on are personal stories or anecdotes. These stories can be very compelling. Many of the therapies highlighted here are those that a number of people found helpful.

As you read through these pages, exercise a healthy skepticism. As mentioned in chapter 4, the placebo effect (an improvement in symptoms even when the substance had no medicinal properties) is very strong in chronic diseases like arthritis. It remains unclear how much people are improving from complementary therapies because those therapies actually work or because of the placebo effect. And until more placebo-controlled clinical studies are done, we will not be able to say for sure.

Communicating with Your Healthcare Provider

If you decide to use a complementary therapy, mention it to your healthcare provider; don't assume you will be asked. The Eisenberg team reported that physicians learn of only 40 percent of the complementary therapies their patients are using. Many healthcare providers don't bring up the topic during an office visit. The Eisenberg team described the current situation as "Don't ask, don't tell."

But communication is important for a number of reasons. Perhaps most important of all is the possibility that a complementary therapy may interact adversely with a medication you are taking at the same time.

Another factor to consider is research. Many complementary therapies are currently being evaluated in clinical trials to determine their effectiveness. Your healthcare provider will likely hear the results of such trials long before you do. The news media report only a small portion of the research findings presented at scientific meetings or published in peer-reviewed professional journals, but your healthcare provider is likely to keep current with such reports and may be able to provide an update on which therapies seem to be effective and which are not.

There is also a practical consideration. Some therapies may be covered by your health insurance plan if your healthcare provider refers you to them.

Last but not least, sharing information with your healthcare provider is important for the same reason you sought out complementary therapies to begin with: because you want to do everything possible to remain healthy. The more information your healthcare provider has about your symptoms and your treatments, the better he or she will be able to advise you.

Complementary Therapies for Arthritis: A to Z

What follows is a primer on some of the therapies used by people with arthritis. Those that are included have been reported as valuable by scientific studies or there is anecdotal evidence of an effect.

How to Spot a Hoax

Although many complementary therapies are worth trying, some are useless. The problem is that advertisements for questionable products are often slick and convincing. So how do you spot a hoax? Here are a few helpful guidelines:

1. The product is promoted as a "cure" for arthritis (there is no cure for arthritis).
2. It contains a "secret formula."
3. Claims are made that the product has been "scientifically proven," but you've never heard of the researchers or the institutions mentioned.
4. The advertisements contain plenty of personal stories about how the product works but little or no scientific studies.
5. There is no list of ingredients.
6. The sponsors claim it has no side effects or do not mention them.

Source: The Arthritis Foundation

In addition, such therapies as vitamins and yoga are covered in chapter 12.

Some therapies are not included here, such as bee venom, cat's claw, copper bracelets, deer antler velvet, devil's claw, ginseng, magnets, and shark cartilage extracts, to name just a few. These may be marketed aggressively, but too little evidence exists that they alleviate the symptoms of arthritis.

For more information about the therapies contained in this chapter, you can consult the organizations listed in Appendix A or you can read an excellent book on the subject published by The Arthritis Foundation, *The Arthritis Foundation's Guide to Alternative Therapies*.

Acupuncture

An ancient Chinese practice, acupuncture has become very popular in the United States as a way to relieve pain. Acupuncture involves the insertion of tiny needles into different points in your body to promote health and interfere with pain signals.

Although you might think that the needles are inserted in or around nerves, which help communicate pain, that is not the case. Acupuncture is based on the Chinese view of the body, in which a life energy known as *qi* (pronounced *chee*) flows through special channels known as meridians. The needles are inserted either to promote the flow of *qi* or to redirect it.

Western medicine does not recognize the existence of *qi* or meridian channels, but we do have some theories about why acupuncture seems to work. It may be that the insertion of needles stimulates the release of endorphins, chemicals that relieve pain, or other hormones and chemicals that dull the pain or at least your perception of it.

Whatever the mechanism, acupuncture does appear to work (at least for some people). A number of studies have reported that it is effective in alleviating arthritis pain. For some people the relief is immediate; for others it takes a few sessions. If you have tried other therapies for your pain and are not receiving adequate relief, you may want to give acupuncture a try.

Aloe

Aloe is derived from the leaves of a type of lily. It is marketed in everything from first aid creams to skin lotions. It can soothe the pain of scrapes and minor burns, and seems to promote healing. You may find it helpful to apply a topical gel or lotion containing aloe to your sore joints. These preparations are available in most pharmacies.

Avocado and Soybean Unsaponifiables (ASU)

DOSAGE: 300 MILLIGRAMS PER DAY

It may surprise you to know that combining two ingredients found in the grocery store could help alleviate your arthritis pain. We certainly were skeptical when we first heard of this approach, but early studies report it may help some people with osteoarthritis. Some theorize ASU may promote cartilage repair, but much more research needs to be done.

ASU is made from one-third avocado oil and two-thirds soybean oil. It is available in pill form in France (where it was first tested) and some countries in Europe, sold under the brand name *Plascledine 300*. (We could not find it in the United States, but you may want to check your local health food store.)

Ayurveda

An ancient Hindu philosophy of healing, ayurveda is still practiced in India and in many parts of the world, including the United States. People who practice ayurveda believe that health results when body, soul, and life energy are in balance. To maintain balance it helps to practice yoga and controlled breathing, and eat vegetarian meals, among other things.

If that advice sounds familiar, it should: Your healthcare provider has probably given it to you using slightly different words (exercise, reduce your stress levels, and eat right). Ayurvedic practitioners also use herbs, minerals, and other natural remedies to help spur healing, but you are unlikely to obtain these from your healthcare provider.

It is not easy to find an ayurvedic practitioner in the United States and there are no certification standards for this profession.

Biofeedback

Biofeedback combines relaxation techniques with electronic measurements of temperature, blood pressure, and other physiological functions in order to teach how to reduce stress at will. In many respects, it is similar to meditation (see entry) but it adds an instant feedback element that you may find helpful. A number of studies have reported that biofeedback is helpful in reducing pain and other symptoms of arthritis while increasing the ability to relax and sleep.

Biofeedback can be done in your healthcare provider's office or with the help of a practitioner who specializes in this approach. He or she will attach electronic sensors to your chest or wrist (or whatever part of the body is being measured); these sensors feed information to a computer or some other type of electronic measurement device. Then you'll try some relaxation exercises to slow your breathing and reduce your blood pressure. The electronic device provides instant feedback on whether the techniques are working. If they are not, you can try another technique and see if that is any better.

Biofeedback can help you find a relaxation technique that works for you. The sensors may detect a difference before you do because of the physiological changes that sometimes take place before actual pain reduction does. That early feedback can encourage you to continue practicing so that you will eventually enjoy relief from pain and other symptoms.

Boron

DOSAGE: 1 TO 3 MILLIGRAMS PER DAY

Boron is a mineral found in certain fruits, vegetables, and dried beans. Some studies report that it can alleviate pain and other symptoms of arthritis. If you eat enough fruits and vegetables (the FDA recommends five servings per day), then you are probably digesting adequate amounts of boron. If not, you may consider taking a boron supplement (but take no more than 3 milligrams per day because women who exceed that amount may increase their estrogen levels). Many multivitamins also contain boron, so check the label if you take a multivitamin before investing in another supplement.

Boswellia

DOSAGE: 150 MILLIGRAMS THREE TIMES A DAY

Boswellia, also known as frankincense, comes from an Asian tree. It is used in India to treat arthritis, and many people find it eases pain. Studies have been mixed, however. It probably won't hurt you if you want to give it a try, but stop using it if you experience nausea or diarrhea, or develop a rash.

Breathing Techniques

Breathing is something we take for granted and may not pay much attention to. But there are ways that you can control your breathing and literally slow it down. That's important because when you are in pain, you may find yourself taking hard, short intakes of breath as you tense up in response to the pain. This only exacerbates the situation. If you can learn to breathe more slowly and deeply, you may find that your pain decreases.

A number of clinical studies have shown this to be the case. For instance, one study reported that people with rheumatoid arthritis who practiced relaxation techniques and other coping mechanisms suffered less pain and anxiety. Another found that children with juvenile rheumatoid arthritis felt less pain after learning breathing techniques and other relaxation strategies.

Most of us are shallow breathers, though we probably don't know it. To learn how to breathe more deeply, try the following steps:

1. Sit in a comfortable position or lie down.
2. Place your hand on your chest and take a deep breath. Your hand should move outward as your chest expands.

3. Now place your hand on your abdomen, just above your waist. Take another breath. Your hand should move. If not, try breathing again and forcing the air downward.
4. Place your hand just below your waist, at the lowest part of your abdomen, and breathe again. Practice breathing until this hand moves as well.

To get the benefits of this method, try to continue deep breathing for several minutes at first and then work up to a ten-minute session. You don't have to take huge breaths to notice the difference; the "deep" here refers to the fact that you take breath deep into your body. Try breathing normally but visualize the air traveling down into the lowest part of your abdomen. And as you exhale, let your body go limp and relax to enhance the effect.

Cartilage-building Substances

A number of cartilage-building products are promoted in health food stores, including cow and shark cartilage as well as supplements like chondroitin sulfate and glucosamine (see entries below). Although there have been some intriguing early studies, there is as yet no firm evidence that taking any type of supplement will actually rebuild or repair cartilage. The process of cartilage degradation and repair is a complicated one, and it changes as we age. This is one area where it makes sense to be a skeptical consumer. (See chapter 2 for more information on cartilage.)

Chinese Medicine

As with ayurveda, Chinese medicine is a philosophy that health results from a balance of key elements. In Chinese medicine the challenge is to balance vital life energies known as yin (that which is cool and passive) and yang (that which is warm and energetic). A related challenge is to keep another life energy, known as *qi* (pronounced *chee*), flowing through the body.

According to this philosophy, illness results when the yin and yang are out of balance and the flow of *qi* has either slowed or stopped altogether. To restore balance and health, you undergo acupuncture (see entry) or use gentle exercises such as *qi gong* (see chapter 12).

Although practitioners of Chinese medicine are not licensed in the United States, many states do certify acupuncturists. For more information see Appendix A.

Acupuncture is probably the best studied aspect of Chinese medicine. Two movement therapies, tai chi and *qi gong* (see chapter 12), also provide some evidence of usefulness.

Chiropractic Medicine

If you have neck and back pain because of arthritis, you may want to visit a chiropractor. These practitioners manipulate and realign vertebrae in the spine and sometimes manipulate other joints as well. This approach is based on the belief that when the spine is out of alignment, it adversely affects the central nervous system (since all nerves eventually lead to the spinal column), causing pain and other damage.

Although many people find chiropractic medicine helpful in reducing pain and restoring movement, researchers have found mixed results. One preliminary study reported that chiropractic techniques relieved pain and improved flexibility in twenty-one people with fibromyalgia, but another study showed that chiropractic manipulations were no better at relieving back pain than physical therapy.

If you have ankylosing spondylitis, osteoporosis, or rheumatoid arthritis, it is best to avoid chiropractic manipulation because it can harm your joints if done too forcefully. On the other hand, if you have a mild to moderate form of arthritis and have not sustained much joint damage (especially in your neck and back), you may find chiropractic manipulation helpful. In any event, it's best to talk with your healthcare provider before making a decision.

Chondroitin Sulfate

DOSAGE: 600 MILLIGRAMS TWO TIMES A DAY

Chondroitin sulfate is one of the components of cartilage (see chapter 2). Some people find that taking this as a supplement (often combined with glucosamine—see entry) eases arthritis pain. Europeans have used it for years.

The theory is that chondroitin inhibits the synthesis of enzymes that destroy cartilage. Clinical studies have had mixed results, and there is as yet no evidence that this supplement helps repair cartilage. Large clinical trials of chondroitin and glucosamine supplements are now being conducted in the United States and Europe.

If you decide to try chondroitin sulfate, you will have to be patient. It can take a month before you know if it works for you. If you don't see any improvement after a month, you can try switching brands because different manufacturers include different amounts of chondroitin in their products.

Also, a word of caution: Read the ingredients carefully. Most chondroitin supplements are made from cattle trachea, but some are made from shark cartilage. Taking too much shark cartilage may put you at risk of contamination by heavy metals that the fish ingested.

Collagen

Collagen is a component of cartilage and of many tissues in our bodies, including skin. Some early studies have reported that a specific type of collagen (type II) may be helpful in easing the pain and inflammation of rheumatoid arthritis, but the effect seems to vary by person and type of collagen used. Other larger, randomized studies have reported that collagen supplements are no more effective than a placebo.

Evening Primrose Oil

DOSAGE: 1.8 GRAMS (1,800 MILLIGRAMS) OF GLA PER DAY

Evening primrose, a weed, contains an omega-6 fatty acid known as gamma-linolenic acid, or GLA. When you digest GLA, you convert it into a substance that reduces inflammation. Several studies have reported that GLA supplements reduce pain and inflammation in people with rheumatoid arthritis and have enabled many of them to reduce their dosage of NSAIDs.

The problem is that you have to take a lot of evening primrose oil supplements (as many as forty capsules a day) to obtain enough GLA to feel any effect. Read the label to see how much GLA your supplement contains (typically each capsule contains about 45 milligrams).

Another precaution: Evening primrose oil can thin your blood, thereby increasing the effects of NSAIDs and other medications. Talk with your healthcare provider before taking this supplement, especially if you are on warfarin *(Coumadin)* or other blood thinners.

An alternative to evening primrose oil is borage oil, which contains more GLA per capsule.

Fish Oil

DOSAGE: 3 GRAMS (3,000 MILLIGRAMS) OF EPA-DHA PER DAY

Fish oil may decrease the inflammation and pain of rheumatoid arthritis, according to early studies. It may be helpful because it contains two omega-3 fatty acids, eicosapentaenoic acid (EPA) and docosahexaenoic acid (DHA), which reduce inflammation.

You can consume more omega-3 fatty acids by eating certain nuts and cold water fish such as mackerel and salmon. Or you can take fish oil supplements available at your local health food store. Some people complain of a fish taste after taking these pills, especially if they are taking quite a few a day.

And as safe as fish might sound, it does have risks for some people. It can thin the blood, so if you are already taking blood thinners, such as aspirin or warfarin *(Coumadin)*, you may end up harming yourself. And because of its blood-thinning effects, fish oil can intensify the side effects of NSAIDs. You may also gain weight because some of the supplements and the food that contain EPA and DHA are high in calories. It is best to talk with your healthcare provider first.

Good Sources of Omega-3 Fatty Acids

Source	Grams per 3.5 ounce serving
Sardines packed in oil	21.1
Dried white walnuts	8.7
Black walnuts	3.3
Green soybeans	3.2
Mackerel	2.5
Herring	1.7
Trout	1.6
Anchovy	1.4
Sablefish	1.4
Salmon	1.2
Bluefish	1.2
Mullet	1.1

Data derived from Judith Horstman, *The Arthritis Foundation's Guide to Alternative Therapies* (Atlanta, Ga.: The Arthritis Foundation, 1999).

Flaxseed

DOSAGE: 1 TO 3 TABLESPOONS OF FLAXSEED OIL OR
1/4 CUP OF FLAXSEED MEAL

Flaxseed is derived from a common plant, but it contains an omega-3 oil that, when digested, is converted into one of the ingredients of fish oil (see page 266). Because flaxseed is available in both oil and solid form, you can add it to your meals fairly easily. You can add it to salad dressing, sprinkle it on food, or mix it in flour when baking something. Flaxseed oil is also available in capsule form.

Clinical studies of flaxseed in treating arthritis are inconclusive, but the fact that some of its ingredients are converted into helpful fatty acids is promising. Flaxseed does not have any serious side effects, so you may want to give it a try. Start with small amounts because too much flaxseed may cause gas or loose bowel movements.

Ginger

DOSAGE: ONE TEASPOON OF FRESH GINGERROOT
STEEPED IN HOT WATER

This common spice derived from the root aids digestion, and some laboratory studies report that it may also alleviate inflammation and pain. Its effect on arthritis is unclear, but using ginger in small doses in tea or in cooking can't hurt. Don't overdo it, though: Too much ginger can cause gastrointestinal upset.

Glucosamine

DOSAGE: 750 MILLIGRAMS TWO TIMES A DAY
OR 500 MILLIGRAMS THREE TIMES A DAY

Glucosamine is a component of cartilage, along with chondroitin. (See chapter 2 for more information about cartilage.) It enhances the synthesis of proteins that build cartilage. In the past few years the supplement glucosamine has been promoted as an arthritis "cure." It is not, but some early studies (and many people) have reported that it eases the pain of osteoarthritis.

Glucosamine, made from crab, lobster, and shrimp shells, is often combined with chondroitin sulfate and sold as supplements (see entry for Chondroitin Sulfate). You may have to take this supplement for a month before noticing any changes in symptoms. If it does not work after a month, you could try another brand. Ingredients vary widely among different manufacturers, so it could be that you are not getting enough of the supplement to notice any effect.

Early studies have reported that glucosamine may actually prevent further joint damage by protecting cartilage. Large clinical studies are now under way in Europe and the United States to determine the effect of both glucosamine and chondroitin sulfate supplements on disease progression. For instance, a $6 million study on the use of glucosamine in treating osteoarthritis is currently under way by the National Institutes of Health and should answer questions about this product.

Green Tea

DOSAGE: THREE TO FOUR CUPS A DAY

Green tea has been used to promote health for thousands of years in China and Japan. Lately it has become popular in the United States as well.

There are interesting preliminary studies on animals with arthritis, which suggest that green tea may reduce the severity of arthritis.

Green tea contains polyphenols, chemicals that behave like antioxidants, which protect cells. Polyphenols may also help reduce inflammation. Although more research needs to be done to determine if green tea can help people with rheumatoid arthritis, certainly drinking this kind of tea can't hurt. Just be aware that green tea contains caffeine, so look for a decaffeinated version if that is a concern for you.

Herbal Remedies

An herb is a plant used as a spice for food or as a medicine. Herbs have been used for thousands of years by Chinese and Indian healers to treat illness and promote health.

Herbs can be used in multiple ways. Dried and fresh herbs can be sprinkled on foods or steeped in hot water to make tea. Health food stores sell herb extracts in capsules or as tinctures.

There is little scientific evidence to determine whether herbal remedies are helpful or not because they have not been studied extensively. (St. John's wort, sometimes used as an antidepressant, is one exception.) Because they are not regulated as drugs are, you should be skeptical of any claims made on a commercial package. As always, talk with your healthcare provider before taking any type of herbal remedy.

If you are pregnant or planning to get pregnant, do not take herbal supplements. Most of them have not been tested on pregnant women, so their effects on the developing fetus are unknown.

The herbal remedies we've included in this work are aloe, boswellia, evening primrose oil, flaxseed, ginger, green tea, kava, stinging nettle, and turmeric.

Homeopathy

To some degree homeopathic practitioners treat disease in the same way that vaccines prevent it: They prod the body into healing itself. A homeopath will ask about your symptoms and then recommend that you take a pill or ointment (available over the counter at your local pharmacy, for the most part) that may temporarily worsen your symptoms and then alleviate them. If the first remedy does not work, he or she will try another, looking for one that will provoke a response.

It is not clear if this approach works or how it works. Some people swear by homeopathy; others find no relief. The studies have produced mixed results.

Hypnosis

This is one of those techniques depicted negatively so often in movies and television that it may seem like a joke or a threat. What may come to mind is the phrase "You are getting sleepy" or an image of someone swinging a watch on a chain back and forth, back and forth.

In fact, hypnosis is closer to meditation or visualization (see entries). If you are susceptible to hypnosis—and anywhere from five to thirty people out of every one hundred are—then it may be a way to reduce the pain of your arthritis.

You can practice self-hypnosis or work with a hypnotist. The process goes something like this:

1. Visualize a peaceful scene to help you relax.
2. If you are working with a hypnotist, he or she will speak in a low, calm voice to help you relax.
3. If you are alone, try counting backward.
4. Gradually, you will be in a state that feels like a trance; you are at peace and open to suggestions.

5. Focus on your goal: relieving pain, gaining more mobility, or merely accepting your arthritis rather than fighting it. Your hypnotist can repeat a phrase to reinforce the goal. If you are alone, you can think about it or repeat a phrase softly to yourself.

A number of studies have reported that hypnosis can be helpful in reducing pain and decreasing stress. It will probably be most useful to you if you use it in conjunction with other relaxation techniques (see entry).

Journal Writing

You've heard about walking off stress, but how about writing it off? An intriguing study reported in 1999 in the *Journal of the American Medical Association* found that nearly half of the people with mild to moderate asthma or rheumatoid arthritis experienced a significant reduction in their symptoms when they took time to write in a journal every day. (Only 24 percent of the control group, who did not write in a journal, improved.) In the study, participants were asked to write about the "most stressful experience in their entire life." They didn't have to write about arthritis—some people wrote about the death of a loved one, for instance—and they didn't have to do it continuously. They wrote for twenty minutes a day for three days.

It's not clear why this technique works. Probably the very act of writing about a bad experience helps people express their emotions about it and thereby relieves stress and anxiety. In any event, journal writing can't hurt, so you may want to give it a try. You may have to be patient to see any results, however. In the study it took four months before any improvement was noticed by the people with rheumatoid arthritis.

Kava

DOSAGE: 140 TO 240 MILLIGRAMS PER DAY

Kava is extracted from the *Piper methysticum* plant that grows in the South Pacific. Drinks made from kava root are soothing, and at least one study has reported that kava decreases anxiety, which in turn can help alleviate pain. You should feel the effect within thirty minutes.

It may be worth a try, but be careful not to drink kava in addition to alcohol or medications that have a sedative effect.

Massage

Massage involves the manipulation, rubbing, and kneading of skin and underlying soft tissues. There are several different types of massage, some more gentle than others and some involving the application of lotions. All types of massage may be effective in loosening tight muscles, reducing pain and soreness, and helping you to relax. You can either visit a professional massage therapist or do it yourself (with your hands or a vibrator).

A few cautions, however. Although massage sounds gentle, it can sometimes involve forceful manipulations, so it's best to talk with your massage therapist beforehand to make sure he or she realizes you have arthritis and your joints may be more tender than those of other clients. And if you are experiencing a flare in your symptoms or your joints are red and inflamed, it is better not to have a massage.

Meditation

Too much to do; too little time. Who hasn't felt that way at least, oh, once a day? As mentioned frequently, if you can reduce your stress level, you will feel less pain from your arthritis and may see other symptoms improve as well. But how to reduce stress when the entire world seems in some kind of mad rush all the time?

Meditation is one technique that you can do anytime and almost anywhere—even in your office (provided you take a few precautions such as turning off the phone and closing the door). Here's how:

1. Find a peaceful, quiet place where you can sit for twenty minutes or a half-hour without being interrupted.
2. Focus on something—a sound, an object, or an image—so that you become less aware of what is around you.

3. Repeat a word or phrase, or listen to a relaxation tape such as the sound of the ocean.
4. Distracting thoughts may occur. If so, let them come and go. Keep repeating a word or phrase.
5. Gradually, you will feel yourself relax.

Experiment with different techniques and see what works for you.

Although the word "meditation" may conjure up an image of an Indian mystic sitting cross-legged on a pillow, you can assume whatever position is comfortable. If your joints are sore, sitting cross-legged may be the last thing you want to do. Sitting in a chair is fine, and so is lying down on a couch or bed (as long as you can stay awake).

If you are experiencing a lot of pain, you may find it difficult to meditate at first. Sometimes sitting quietly only makes you more aware of the throbbing in your joints. Some people try to work through this and find that eventually the relaxation response does decrease their pain. If you cannot bear sitting still, don't. One alternative is to take a quiet walk and do a moving meditation.

A number of studies have reported that meditation decreases pain and anxiety in people with various types of chronic diseases including arthritis. Part of the effect seems to come from the decrease in heart rate, blood pressure, and chemicals associated with stress. Also beneficial is a sense of gaining control over your body, which can seem out of control when you have arthritis. So you may find some benefit from a meditation method that works for you and that you can use every day.

We may learn more in the future. In 1998, Congress added $10 million a year for five years to the budget of the National Institutes of Health so that the agency could increase research and training about the mind-body connection, especially the use of meditation.

Muscle Relaxation

It is also possible to relax particular muscles one at a time or in groups. This technique, known as progressive muscle relaxation, can be done before you try meditation or visualization (see entries).

Muscle relaxation has seldom been studied on its own. One small study reported that eight people with irritable bowel syndrome improved more than a control group after learning progressive muscle relaxation. More often, muscle relaxation has been studied in conjunction with several relaxation methods. One randomized controlled trial reported that relaxation techniques decreased pain and anxiety in people with rheumatoid arthritis.

Progressive muscle relaxation is exactly what it sounds like: You focus on relaxing one muscle group at a time. It is best to start at the top or the bottom of your body. Try the following steps, starting with your neck and shoulders.

1. Raise your head toward the ceiling without going on tiptoe. You should feel a pull in your neck.
2. Hold the position for a few seconds and then relax.
3. Lift your shoulders up to the ceiling.
4. Hold that position for a few seconds and then relax.
5. Make a tight fist.
6. Hold for a few seconds and then relax.
7. Breathe in so that your chest pulls up.
8. Hold that position a few seconds, then exhale slowly.
9. Tense the muscles in your thighs and buttocks.
10. Hold for a few seconds and then relax.
11. Scrunch your toes, as if you were trying to reach backward to your ankle.
12. Hold for a few seconds and then relax.

As you do this exercise, you should notice that your muscles will feel much more at ease once you have flexed and released them. By the end of it you should feel more relaxed than you did before.

If any of your muscles hurt while you are going through this progressive routine, don't hold the position that caused the pain. Instead, try massaging the muscle gently with your hand to help it relax.

Naturopathic Medicine

Naturopathic practitioners, as their name implies, use natural therapies to treat illness. Emphasis is on a good diet, regular exercise, and avoidance of toxins and poisons. The goal is to keep yourself so healthy that you are able to heal yourself.

Some of this may sound familiar; your own healthcare provider has probably recommended the same. However, naturopathic practitioners tend to focus more on changes you can make in your day-to-day life that will help with your symptoms. And because they cannot and do not want to prescribe drugs, naturopathic practitioners rely on herbal remedies, physical therapies, and homeopathy.

There are many naturopathic practitioners in the United States and a number of states license them.

Osteopathic Medicine

Osteopathic practitioners view the musculoskeletal system as the key to health. If your body is out of alignment or your muscles are weak, your health may suffer; likewise, if you become ill, your musculoskeletal system may be affected. To treat illness or help you maintain your health, osteopaths will manipulate the spine, joints, and muscles. The idea is to restore balance so that your body can heal itself.

All fifty states license osteopaths, and they can prescribe medications. In fact, the training of an osteopath is very similar to that of a medical doctor.

Prayer

A number of intriguing studies have reported that prayer can alleviate symptoms of illness, speed healing, and even prolong life. Although many of these studies have been faulted for poor methodology, prayer remains a viable (and popular) complement to standard therapy. As in meditation, you may find that praying helps you relax and alleviates your pain. If you are a spiritual person who believes in God or a higher power, you may benefit by praying.

Relaxation Techniques

Many of the therapies described in this work involve some type of relaxation technique. Hypnosis, Meditation, and Visualization all encourage you to relax. If you are having trouble relaxing or even sitting still, you may need to take it a step further and focus more on your breathing and on the tension in your body. See Breathing Techniques or Muscle Relaxation Techniques.

SAM or SAMe (S-adenosylmethionine)

DOSAGE: 200 TO 400 MILLIGRAMS THREE TIMES A DAY

We make S-adenosylmethionine (SAM) naturally from adenosine triphosphate and an amino acid, methionine. Eating enough green leafy vegetables, which provide folic acid, helps our cells make enough SAM to support a number of biochemical reactions essential to life. Among other things, SAM helps neurotransmitters function, which affects mood, and is one of the chemicals involved in cartilage repair and generation.

SAM supplements (sometimes marketed as SAMe, which is pronounced like the man's name "Sammy"), used for almost twenty years in Europe, have recently become available in this country. These supplements have been promoted as treatments for depression, fibromyalgia, and osteoarthritis. Although a number of studies have been done in Europe, clinical data in this country are scarce. One study in the United States concluded that SAMe supplements may alleviate mild to moderate pain from osteoarthritis. The results of studies on this supplement's effect on fibromyalgia, done in Europe, have been mixed.

If you have rheumatoid arthritis and are taking methotrexate, you should not take SAMe supplements. Methotrexate reduces the levels of SAM in your blood; by taking a SAMe supplement, you could counteract the effect of the drug.

For people with other types of arthritis, the supplements do appear to be safe, but we don't know enough about them yet to recommend them. You should also be aware that these supplements are expensive, costing anywhere from $79 to $210 per month depending on how much you take and what brand you buy.

You may be better off eating more dark leafy green vegetables such as broccoli and lettuce so that you can produce SAM on your own. Or take B vitamins (folic acid and B_{12}), which will help you to better use the SAM you produce on your own.

Stinging Nettle (Also Known as Urtica)

DOSAGE: UNDETERMINED; ONE GERMAN STUDY USED 50 GRAMS OF STEWED *URTICA DIOICA;* ANOTHER USED 1,340 MILLIGRAMS OF *URTICA DIOICA* POWDER.

Some people find stinging nettle helpful in reducing pain and inflammation. Although some herbalists claim that applying dried leaves to a sore joint will ease pain, there is no clinical evidence for this. Two German studies have reported that taking stinging nettle supplements or sprinkling cooked leaves on food may help reduce pain and inflammation and enable you to decrease the dosage of your medications. This herb may be available as a supplement, a dried powder extract, or as dried leaves that can be cooked. (Look for "stinging nettle" or *Urtica dioica.*)

Turmeric

DOSAGE: 400 MILLIGRAMS THREE TIMES A DAY

You may be familiar with turmeric as a spice; it is often used in Indian food. Some people have found that combining turmeric with boswellia and ginger (see entries) helps reduce pain and inflammation. Few clinical studies have been done.

Visualization

Think positive. Who hasn't heard that advice? It may seem ridiculous when so much about arthritis seems negative, but focusing on a "best case scenario" may actually help reduce pain and improve mobility.

Visualization is a way of thinking positive. In many ways it is similar to meditation (see entry). Try the following steps:

1. Sit in a quiet place.
2. Imagine a scene from the life you would like to be living. For instance, if you have osteoarthritis of the knee and have given up basketball, perhaps imagine yourself shooting hoops and intercepting passes with all the skill and ease you had in college. If

you have rheumatoid arthritis that has flared recently, imagine a peaceful country road and see yourself walking without pain.
3. Imagine another scene such as running a marathon, cooking a gourmet meal, or swing dancing—whatever suits your fancy.

Although studies about the effects of visualization have been inconclusive, some people swear by it. When the technique works, it seems to do so by encouraging you to focus on something besides your pain and arthritis. This enables you to relax and breathe more slowly—and you may actually feel less pain as a result. It is worth a try and certainly can't hurt you.

Willow Bark Tea

This beverage may alleviate minor aches and pains. The active ingredient in willow bark tea is salicylic acid, the main ingredient in aspirin. However, you would have to drink a lot of willow bark tea—as many as ten cups—to enjoy the same benefits as two aspirin. And too much tea (like too much aspirin) may upset your stomach.

Zinc Supplements

DOSAGE: 50 MILLIGRAMS OR LESS PER DAY

Some studies have reported that people with rheumatoid arthritis have low levels of zinc. Several early studies reported that taking zinc supplements may help alleviate the symptoms of both rheumatoid arthritis and psoriatic arthritis. Other researchers dispute these findings, however, and the jury is still out. There is no agreement among rheumatologists about whether zinc supplement will help you.

You can take the supplements if you wish, but taking more than 50 milligrams per day may harm you.

Information to Share with Your Healthcare Provider

1. If you are currently using a complementary therapy, tell your healthcare provider about it.

2. Write down the amounts of herbs, vitamins, and other dietary supplements you are taking. Better yet, bring the packages with you.
3. Mention why it is important for you to use complementary therapies and the type of symptoms that prompted you to seek a complementary therapy. This information will help your healthcare provider better understand the challenges of your arthritis.
4. If you have had any positive or adverse results after taking a complementary therapy, mention it to your healthcare provider.

Questions to Ask Your Healthcare Provider

1. How do you feel about complementary or alternative medicines?
2. Do you have any cautions for me based on what I've told you about the therapies I'm using?
3. Do you have any other suggestions for alternative therapies that may be appropriate for my situation?
4. Is there any chance that the supplements I am taking will adversely interact with or affect my medications?
5. What brands of particular supplements do you recommend?
6. Where can I find more information?

CHAPTER 12

Living with Arthritis

What happens if I get pregnant? Should I stop taking my medications? What will happen to my symptoms if I do? What will happen to my baby if I don't?

What changes should I make in my diet and in my exercise routine now that I have arthritis? There is so much conflicting information out there.

Between the pain and the medications, I just don't want to have sex anymore, but I don't want my relationship with my wife to suffer. What do I do?

ARTHRITIS, LIKE any other chronic disease, can alter your life profoundly, often in unexpected ways. Suddenly you may not be able to do things you always took for granted: cooking a meal, body surfing in the ocean with your children, or even making love to your partner. Fortunately, you can modify your habits and improve your overall health so that you will be able to live your life as normally as before.

Eating Well

Although there are plenty of "arthritis diets" being promoted, the best strategy is to eat a healthy, well-balanced diet to maintain your health. Eating exorbitant amounts of a particular food or eliminating others is unlikely to improve your symptoms and may even worsen them.

The components of a healthy diet are detailed in chapter 3, but here are some additional tips to keep in mind:

- Eating five servings per day of fruits and vegetables is even more important when you have arthritis. Your body needs a regular supply of vitamins and minerals to cope with the symptoms of this disease.

• Watch the fat content in foods and try to cut back. Since being overweight will only exacerbate your pain and other symptoms, now is the time to reduce fat intake.

• You may want to add certain foods to your diet such as fish and leafy green vegetables. Some types of fish provide omega-3 fatty acids, which some early studies have found help protect your joints and even ease pain. Leafy green vegetables provide a number of vitamins essential to keeping you healthy.

Vitamin and Mineral Supplements

Although you may think you eat a balanced diet, you still may not be getting enough vitamins and minerals every day. As we get older, we metabolize food differently and may not absorb vitamins as well. Your arthritis may also have profound effects on the way your body burns fuel. And the medications you take for your symptoms may also interfere with vitamin and mineral absorption.

For all these reasons you may want to consider taking a multivitamin supplement that provides adequate amounts of the essential vitamins and minerals without harm. Then take additional supplements if your healthcare provider recommends it.

Why the caution? Some vitamins, such as C, are water soluble, which means that if your body does not use them, they will be excreted. But others, such as vitamin E, are fat soluble. That means your body can store them if it doesn't use them, and they can build up to toxic levels if you overdo it.

To help you understand why certain vitamins are important, here is a brief description.

Vitamin A. Also known as beta-carotene, it has been touted as a preventive agent for everything from aging to cancer. There is some truth to these claims: Vitamin A is an antioxidant, which helps protect cells against "free radicals," highly reactive molecules that roam the body, sometimes inflicting damage. Some studies show that vitamin A slows the progression of joint damage in osteoarthritis. Other studies show it may actually increase the damage, for reasons that are unclear. Although taking beta-carotene was promoted a few years ago, we now recommend that you don't take it as a supplement. It is better for your health to get vitamin A the natural way—by eating plenty of fruits and vegetables.

The B vitamins. There are actually several types of B vitamins, including B_1 (thiamine), B_2 (riboflavin), B_3 (niacin), B_5 (pantothenic acid), B_6 (pyridoxine), and B_{12}. You can find them packaged separately or as a B-complex vitamin (which does not usually include B_{12}). Some studies show B_3 may help reduce the amount of medication needed to control the pain of osteoarthritis; other studies show B_5 helps decrease pain and increase mobility for people with rheumatoid arthritis. (As always, the best person to check with is your healthcare provider.) B_6 and B_{12} are important for overall health.

Vitamin C. Some studies have shown that taking relatively high amounts of vitamin C can reduce the pain and severity of osteoarthritis. The best way to get vitamin C is by eating oranges or other citrus fruits, but supplements are also available. Aim for 500 to 1000 milligrams a day. One note of caution, however: Consuming too much vitamin C can upset your stomach or cause diarrhea.

Vitamin D. We can make this substance on our own, given the right climate and circumstances. When your skin is exposed to sunlight, your body responds by making vitamin D, which helps build and protect bones. The problem, of course, is that most of us don't spend much time outdoors. And we in the United States, spend six months of the year with relatively few hours of sunlight per day.

You can also obtain vitamin D by drinking fortified milk and eating fatty fish. If you don't get enough vitamin D each day, you can take a supplement. An analysis of the ongoing Framingham Heart Study reported that if you consume adequate amounts each day, you may be able to reduce the pain and severity of osteoarthritis. Aim for 400 to 800 IU (international units) per day. Don't take more than that, however; if you take too much, the calcium levels in your blood can reach toxic levels because vitamin D helps your body absorb calcium in your diet.

Vitamin E. This vitamin has received much attention recently for decreasing the risk of heart disease and possibly protecting your brain against Alzheimer's disease. Some early research has also shown that vitamin E may reduce the pain of arthritis, but other research has concluded that certain vitamin E supplements, which contain a substance known as gamma-tocopherol, may actually worsen your arthritis. (Most vitamin E supplements contain alpha-tocopherol.)

Until more is known, it is best not to take too much vitamin E. Try to consume from 400 to 600 IU per day.

In addition to the vitamins listed above, you may also want to consume extra amounts of two essential nutrients: calcium and folic acid.

Calcium helps protect the bones and joints, and promotes overall good health. It can be found naturally in dairy products, canned fish such as sardines, and leafy green vegetables. Or you can take a supplement, which is especially important if you are a woman because after menopause you will begin to lose bone mass in the process known as osteoporosis unless you do something to prevent it. Aim for 1,000 to 1,500 milligrams per day, depending on your age and whether you are taking any medications. Even adolescents and young women should take calcium supplements to build bone mass before menopause occurs. Typical brand names of calcium supplements include *Citrical, Caltrate,* and *Tums.*

Our cells need folic acid in order to function, and folic acid helps our bodies produce S-adenosylmethionine, a nutrient that keeps cartilage healthy. Folic acid supplements are very important if you are taking methotrexate because folic acid reduces the side effects of this medication. Folic acid is also important if you are pregnant or planning to become pregnant. Check with your healthcare provider first, but as a general rule, aim for 1 milligram of folic acid per day.

Protect Your Joints

Once you have arthritis, you need to do two things simultaneously: put less pressure on your joints and provide more support.

Although splints and orthotics provide one option (see chapter 10), you can also protect your joints on your own during the course of your everyday activities. Sometimes this is a matter of changing the way you do things or making adaptations to your environment. A few simple tips will help you get through your day while putting less strain on your joints:

- If your feet hurt after wearing a particular pair of shoes, try padded insoles (available in any pharmacy and in many department stores). This is a cheap way of "adapting" your shoes to provide greater support.
- Wrap large rubber bands around doorknobs; this will make it easier to grip and turn them.
- Buy a small timer for your office and set it to go off every thirty to sixty minutes. This will remind you to get up and stretch regularly. (You can put it in a drawer to muffle the sound if you want.)
- A piece of rubber mesh will make it easier to open jars or grip small objects such as pens and cooking utensils. It is often available in the shelf liner section of a hardware or department store.
- Sleep with an electric blanket, preferably with a timer set to go off an hour before you rise. You will be less stiff if you warm your joints and muscles before getting up in the morning.
- Get a vertical file for your desk top at work to hold current files. That way you won't have to bend to go through file drawers.
- Wear gloves while you garden; this will not only protect your hands but also make it easier to grip gardening tools.

You can also buy products designed to help you do certain activities with less pressure on your joints—anything from opening a bottle to working on a computer. Here are some products that will make your life easier:

- Headset telephones enable you to talk without gripping the receiver for prolonged periods of time. A cordless version will enable you to move about at the same time.
- Ergonomically designed products such as keyboards, staplers, scissors, and key rings make it easier to perform a

task with less pressure. For instance, the Orbit Key Ring (available at www.solutionscatalog.com) enables you to remove or add keys by pressing a stainless steel ball.

- Sneakers with Velcro closures make it possible to avoid shoelaces. Or you can "adapt" your sneakers by buying a Velcro closure to replace the shoelaces (see www.speedstrap.com).
- If you have trouble with your computer mouse, a number of vendors offer "touch pad" devices that move the cursor with less strain on your hand. For example, see the Cirque Cruise Cat at www.cirque.com.

Exercising with Arthritis

Exercise has been shown to decrease pain and increase mobility in people with arthritis. It is one of the best things you can do for yourself to prevent disability and can also improve your cardiovascular health. Few people realize just how dangerous a sedentary lifestyle can be. Some experts believe that inactivity and sedentary living are as risky to your health as smoking a pack of cigarettes a day.

But when it comes to exercise and arthritis, you may feel as if you are being faced with a "chicken and egg" situation. How can you reduce your pain through exercise when you're in so much pain you don't want to move?

Some of this has been covered in chapter 10 on physical therapy. The best strategy is to take non-exercise steps to reduce pain (such as medication or joint rest and bracing) and then begin an exercise routine slowly, focusing on strengthening muscles, improving flexibility by stretching muscles, and improving cardiovascular fitness through aerobic exercises. Work with a physical therapist to develop a tailored exercise plan that will meet your particular needs and ensure that you don't overdo it.

In addition, there are some things you can do for yourself at home—such as playing a video on your home VCR. The Arthritis Foundation has produced several excellent exercise videos. You can actually go through a fitness routine while watching how the exercises are done. (And who hasn't wanted to put an exercise routine on "pause" occasionally while you catch your breath?) These tapes can be ordered through the Arthritis Foundation, borrowed from a local chapter, or may even be available at your local library.

Other exercise videos for people with arthritis are available at your local bookstore or through online services such as www.amazon.com and www.bn.com. Some suggestions:

- *Exercise Can Beat Arthritis,* a system of gentle low-impact exercises
- *Tai Chi for Arthritis,* a good introduction to tai chi

Available from the Arthritis Foundation at www.arthritis.org:

- *Pathways to Better Living with Arthritis and Related Conditions* includes breathing techniques, stretching and strengthening exercises, and low-impact endurance activities.
- *Keep FIT with Fibromyalgia* will teach you how to manage your pain and stiffness while improving your fitness.
- *PACE: People with Arthritis Can Exercise* is two separate tapes with stretching, strengthening, and endurance exercises.
- *PEP: Pool Exercise Program* is a good way to learn how to exercise in the water.

Explore Other Forms of Exercise

To keep moving and active you may also want to try other exercises that are particularly useful for people with arthritis such as the following which are easy on the joints and good for overall fitness.

Alexander Technique

The Alexander technique is one of several programs that teach you how to move and hold your body differently so that your pain as well as the strain on your joints is reduced. It is named for its creator, F. Mathias Alexander, an actor.

To learn the technique properly, you must take lessons with a certified practitioner (your healthcare provider or physical therapist may be able to provide a referral). Much of the time is spent teaching you how to become aware of how to sit, stand, and walk properly. That may sound absurd, but if you are in pain, chances are you are compensating with another part of your body in order to alleviate the pain. For instance, you may be putting too much strain on your right knee to spare your arthritic left knee. The Alexander technique involves making you more aware of how you currently move and stand, and then making you aware of how you should carry yourself.

Few studies have been done about the Alexander technique, but what few data exist suggest that it may be of use. It may require a significant time and money commitment, however. Typically, people take thirty or more lessons before they can perform the movements on their own.

Feldenkrais Method

In some respects the Feldenkrais method is similar to the Alexander technique. The goal is to make you more aware of how you move and carry yourself, and then teach you better posture so that you can reduce the strain on your joints. The method is named for Moshe Feldenkrais who developed it while recovering from a knee injury.

The Feldenkrais method not only teaches you how to carry yourself better, but it also provides a series of range-of-motion and flexibility movements. Less vigorous than exercise, these movements generally focus on one set of muscles at a time. Some movements are performed while lying down, others while sitting or standing.

There is little scientific data about the Feldenkrais method. If you are willing to invest a fair amount of time (lessons can last for six weeks), this may be worth looking into. Your healthcare provider or physical therapist should be able to refer you to a local practitioner.

Tai Chi

People performing tai chi movements may look as if they are dancing; these exercises are slow and fluid, one leading into the next. Oddly enough, the practice evolved from the martial arts and involves many motions similar to karate—just done at a slow pace and with peaceful intent.

Carry Tiger, Push Mountain

Tai chi resembles a slow-motion dance, but the names of individual movements may remind you of poetry. Carry Tiger, Push Mountain *is a beginner movement, meant to build balance and flexibility.*

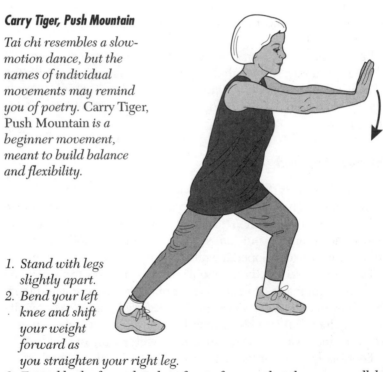

1. *Stand with legs slightly apart.*
2. *Bend your left knee and shift your weight forward as you straighten your right leg.*
3. *Extend both of your hands in front of you so that they are parallel to your shoulder.*
4. *Now lower your arms slowly so that your hands face down, while keeping your legs in the same position as before.*

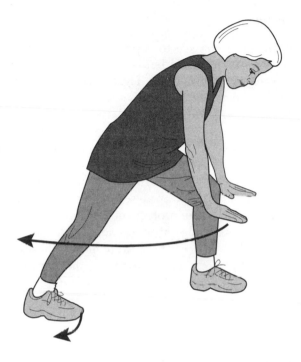

Tai chi, which originated in China, is intended to enable a life force known as *qi* to flow through the body. *Qi* has no Western equivalent but is the basis of a number of complementary therapies, including acupuncture.

Many community centers offer classes in tai chi. A typical session lasts about an hour. You'll first do deep-breathing and gentle stretching exercises. Then you will go through a series of poses that have names like Part the Wild Horse's Mane and Golden Rooster Stands on One Leg. (Many of these movements originated from watching animals in the wild.) See above for an example.

There have been few clinical studies on tai chi conducted in the West, but what few there are indicate that it is safe for people with arthritis and may help decrease pain and increase balance and mobility. It is worth a try.

Trager Approach

The Trager approach seeks to imprint new patterns of movement in your brain so that you will both consciously and unconsciously change the way you carry yourself. The technique was developed by Milton Trager, a doctor and former boxer.

In a Trager session, a therapist will ask that you lie down on a work table while he or she gently moves various parts of your body. The idea is to show you that movement can be pleasant rather than painful and to provide tips on how to move differently so that you will not experience as much pain. In other sessions you may actually go through range-of-motion exercises to become more aware of your body and how to better protect your joints.

There is scant scientific evidence about whether the Trager approach is useful, but it doesn't appear to hurt. Typically, you might need four to eight sessions in order to master the new movements.

Qi Gong

Qi (pronounced *chee*) *gong* is in many respects similar to tai chi. It is intended to improve the flow of the life energy *qi* through the body. The Chinese believe this helps promote good health and cure illness.

However, *qi gong* involves far fewer motions than tai chi, which are done as separate movements interspersed with pauses rather than one long, fluid sequence. For that reason you may find it easier to do *qi gong* if you have moderate to severe arthritis since you will be able to rest briefly before starting the next movement.

As with tai chi, a typical session begins with deep breathing and gentle warm-up exercises. The idea is to quiet your mind as well as your body so you can become attuned to the flow of your *qi*. Then you undertake a series of postures one at a time.

Few studies about the effectiveness of *qi gong* have been conducted in the West, but what data exist suggest that this practice may help reduce your pain and improve mobility. And since *qi gong* involves fewer movements than tai chi, it may be a good way to become familiar with this approach to healing.

Yoga

Yoga originated in India but has become very popular in the United States as a way of improving muscle strength and flexibility and reducing stress. But yoga is actually as much a philosophy as it is a physical practice. It is a way to better unite body, mind, and spirit.

One of the many benefits of yoga, especially if you have arthritis, is that the movements and positions are gentle and can be done at your own pace. You can learn how to do yoga by watching a video, but if

Sample Yoga Asanas

Yoga positions or asanas *are often named for animals or elements in nature. Sometimes the position resembles its namesake, as seen in these illustrations. But each asana is also intended to awaken your appreciation for the environment and all living things that dwell in it, as well as make you more flexible.*

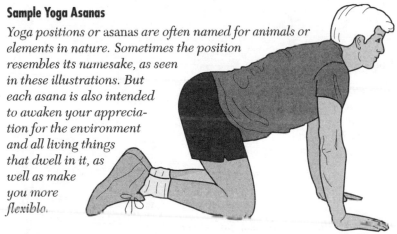

Cat

This asana will improve the flexibility of your spine and firm stomach muscles.

1. *Kneel and lean forward so that your thighs and arms are at a 90-degree angle to the floor.*
2. *As you inhale, point your chin and tailbone up, reaching for the sky.*
3. *Exhale slowly as you tuck under your chin and arch your back, contracting your stomach muscles at the same time.*
4. *Hold a few seconds.*
5. *Repeat entire motion two more times.*

you are new to it, you may consider taking a class. Almost every town offers classes in yoga nowadays, and the cost is usually reasonable.

A typical yoga class lasts an hour. You'll do deep-breathing exercises and gentle stretching exercises. Then you will assume a series of yoga poses, or asanas, which are designed to improve flexibility, balance, and strength. See below for some examples.

Only a few well designed clinical studies have been done about yoga, but they indicate that it can reduce pain and improve mobility, while also reducing stress and anxiety. But anecdotal evidence about the benefits of yoga is strong, and for the most part yoga is safe if you have arthritis. You may want to talk with your healthcare provider before taking a class to find out if there are any poses you should avoid.

Frog

*Another exercise that improves
spinal mobility is the frog asana.
This is similar to the cat asana
described above, but you perform
the movement while seated.*

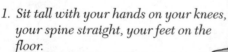

1. *Sit tall with your hands on your knees,
   your spine straight, your feet on the
   floor.*
2. *Lean forward slightly and arch
   your back, inhaling as you do so.
   Point your chin toward the ceiling.*
3. *Hold for several seconds.*
4. *Exhale slowly as you tuck under your chin and round your back,
   still holding onto your knees.*
5. *Hold for several seconds.*
6. *Repeat sequence two more times.*

Tree

This asana will make you more flexible and improve your balance. It may take some practice. Be sure to hold onto something for balance; to avoid a fall, do this barefoot (less likely to slip than socks).

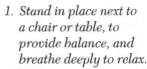

1. Stand in place next to a chair or table, to provide balance, and breathe deeply to relax.
2. Pick a point on the wall to hold your gaze, which will help you to maintain your balance.
3. Slowly raise your right leg off the floor and rest the bottom of your right foot on the inside of your left knee, with your right knee turned out at a 90-degree angle. Breathe normally as you do so.
4. Now raise your right arm over your head, keeping your shoulders level.
5. Hold the pose and your breath for several seconds.
6. Exhale and slowly lower your right arm and leg.
7. Repeat sequence with your left arm and leg.

A variation on this asana is to lift both arms up, as if you were getting ready to dive into a pool, instead of lifting just one arm at a time. But it's best to start with one arm and then progress to two once your balance is sufficiently improved.

Pregnancy and Arthritis

If you are a woman of childbearing age who has arthritis, you may be thinking about whether you should become pregnant. Will you pass the condition onto your baby? Should you go off whatever medications you are taking? And if you do, will you suffer a flare of symptoms because of it?

There are no simple answers when it comes to arthritis and pregnancy, and relatively few studies have looked at the issue. Nevertheless, what we do know is encouraging. By taking a few precautions and working with your general healthcare provider or rheumatologist as well as your obstetrician, you should be able to enjoy a normal pregnancy and give birth to a healthy child.

The one exception to this general rule is Lyme disease, which can be passed on to your baby unless you are treated. It is important to mention if you are pregnant—or trying to become so—when you visit your healthcare provider for treatment of Lyme disease. Although you may still be given antibiotics, they may be administered by injection rather than in pill form.

The good news, which you may find surprising, is that for many women the symptoms of arthritis actually disappear or subside during pregnancy. This issue has been studied most in rheumatoid arthritis. Various studies have found that three out of four pregnant women will see their rheumatoid arthritis symptoms subside, some during their first trimester and a quarter during their second or third trimester.

Once the baby is born, however, the disease generally returns and is as bad as it was before. This generally happens within the first two months after delivery, but it may take longer for some women.

Why Pregnancy Is Protective

So what is going on? The short answer is: We're not sure why being pregnant seems to alleviate symptoms in many women. Some studies suggest that hormonal changes and increases in certain proteins, which occur during pregnancy, may be at work, but this has not been confirmed.

Other investigations have suggested that the fetus may actually protect the mother during pregnancy, in part because the fetus has a different genetic makeup. But thus far we have not been able to determine or duplicate the mechanisms involved. Much more research in this area needs to be done.

In the meantime, if you have arthritis and want to become pregnant, talk with your healthcare provider. One word of caution, though: Do not become pregnant in order to ease your symptoms. It doesn't work for every woman, and it certainly isn't a good reason to become pregnant.

Will I Pass My Arthritis on to My Child?

This is a common concern among women with arthritis. Although some types of arthritis run in families, the rules governing heredity are complicated and still under investigation.

We do know that certain genes are associated with particular types of arthritis. For example, the gene B-27 is associated with the development of ankylosing spondylitis. However, having these genes does not mean that you will develop it. It's important to remember that genes are inherited, but the disease itself is not.

Medications and Pregnancy

There is one area that requires extra caution if you want to become pregnant: medications. Some are safe for you and your baby, others are not. And it may take weeks, even months, for your body to rid itself of some of the medications that could cause birth defects. There are shortcuts in some cases. The best bet is to talk with your healthcare provider if you are even considering becoming pregnant.

Antibiotics. There are certain antibiotics that you should not take while pregnant, including those in the tetracycline family, doxycycline being among them. Please check with your healthcare provider before taking an antibiotic.

Aspirin. Stop taking aspirin when you become pregnant. It can increase your risk of bleeding and hemorrhage, both during pregnancy and after childbirth.

NSAIDs and COX-2 inhibitors. You should stop taking these when you are pregnant. Animal studies have shown that NSAIDs do not increase the chance of birth defects. However, we remain cautious about these medications during pregnancy. Talk with your rheumatologist about alternatives to NSAIDs if you want to become pregnant.

Corticosteroids. You can continue to take corticosteroids while pregnant. Occasionally, if you are taking high doses, your baby may need to receive a supplement of the drug after you deliver.

Disease-modifying anti-rheumatic drugs. DMARDS generally should not be used during pregnancy.

Methotrexate. This medication may cause birth defects if taken at the time of conception or during pregnancy. If you stop taking methotrexate for at least one menstrual cycle before trying to conceive, you will avoid this risk.

Sulfasalazine. This is one of the few DMARDs that you can use if you are pregnant. However, you should use it with caution, especially during the final months of pregnancy. Talk with your rheumatologist before making a decision.

Leflunomide. Leflunomide (see page 162), marketed under the brand name *Arava,* can cause birth defects. It also remains in your body long after you have taken the last pill. If you are taking the medication currently but want to have a child, speak with your rheumatologist. He or she can best advise you how to come off the drug and how to eliminate it from your body, and when it will be safe to conceive.

Herbal Remedies and Pregnancy

If you are pregnant or thinking of becoming pregnant, you should also stop taking herbal supplements. (Herbal teas are fine.) Many supplements contain relatively large amounts of herbs and may contain other products. Not many products considered dietary supplements have been tested at all, never mind in pregnant women, so we have no way of knowing how they might affect your fetus. It is therefore better not to use them while you are pregnant.

Pay Special Attention to Diet

You must pay special attention to diet while you are pregnant if you have arthritis. You can become anemic because of an iron or folic acid deficiency. If you have rheumatoid arthritis, your risk is even greater because the disease commonly results in both iron deficiency and folic acid deficiency.

During pregnancy you transfer iron to your baby and the placenta, and you may need as much as ten times the iron you normally would. You should therefore talk with your healthcare provider and/or obstetrician about taking iron supplements.

Folic acid needs also increase during pregnancy, partly because you are less able to absorb it and partly because so much of it goes to the fetus. Supplemental folic acid is essential to prevent certain birth defects. Talk with your obstetrician about how much of these supplements you should take.

Protecting Your Joints While Pregnant

Although some types of arthritis actually ease up during pregnancy, in other cases you may find your symptoms worsen. This is especially true if you have arthritis in your weight-bearing joints such as your knees and hips. For starters, you gain weight during pregnancy and this places increased pressure on your joints. As you progress to full term, you will have more difficulty walking and holding an erect posture, which only compounds the problems.

Fortunately, there are steps you can take to protect your joints during pregnancy. The following are based on recommendations by the Arthritis Foundation.

1. Eat a good diet that supplies nutrients but does not add pounds unrelated to your pregnancy.

2. Keep exercising. This may be the time to take up water aerobics or to ask your healthcare provider about isometric exercises in which you tense the muscle without moving the joint.
3. Talk to your healthcare provider or therapist about orthotic devices for your shoes to provide more support.
4. Try wearing support hosiery. This will help support your joints and also minimize fluid retention in your legs and ankles.
5. Wear running shoes all the time. Available at any sporting goods store, they provide much more support than ordinary shoes.
6. Take frequent rests or time-outs. Sit down and literally "take a load off" your hips, knees, and ankles.
7. If your joints hurt, try applying heat or cold to the area in order to avoid taking medications. (See chapter 10.)
8. You can also try some deep-breathing and relaxation exercises. The more relaxed you are, the less intensely you will feel pain.
10. A firm mattress will provide support to your joints and prevent you from aching in the morning.

Labor and Delivery

Most women with arthritis are able to deliver their babies vaginally. One area of concern, of course, is all the pressure placed on your joints during labor. This will be an issue if your arthritis affects your hips, pelvis, or spine.

Some women have used special birthing seats to help support their hips and legs, enabling them to sit up rather than lie down. Or you might find it easier to lie on your side.

If this is a concern, discuss the issue with your obstetrician and/or healthcare provider in advance.

Postpartum Issues

Unfortunately, you may face several challenges once you have given birth. All can be dealt with, but it is better to be aware of them in advance.

If your symptoms have gone into remission during pregnancy, they are likely to return once you have given birth. In one study, 81 percent of women with rheumatoid arthritis who had gone into remission during pregnancy had their symptoms return in the postpartum period. It is important to talk with your rheumatologist as well as your obstetrician about the steps you can take to alleviate these symptoms. You may return to the medications you were taking before.

Not surprisingly, the return of symptoms (and the hormonal changes typical of the postpartum period) can cause depression and may also add to the fatigue you feel from caring for a new baby. You can cope with some of these effects on your own, using some of the complementary therapies discussed in chapter 11. The first thing to do is talk with your healthcare provider about changes to your diet because some of these symptoms may be due to anemia and poor eating habits.

Certainly, if you continue to feel depressed, you and your healthcare provider should discuss medications. Many are available that can provide relief fairly quickly.

Breast-feeding and Arthritis

Breast-feeding is good for your baby, but the situation gets complicated if you have arthritis. For starters, there is a chance that you will pass on to your baby some of the medications you are taking.

There is also a risk if you have rheumatoid arthritis that you will exacerbate your arthritis. It's not clear why breast-feeding would be a risk to you. One study suggested that women with severe rheumatoid arthritis had breast-fed more children and for longer periods of time than those with mild to moderate forms of the disease. Some studies suggest that the hormone prolactin, which encourages milk secretion, may also encourage inflammation.

Although more research needs to be done, you may want to consider breast-feeding carefully before deciding what you will do. Talk it over with your rheumatologist as well as your obstetrician.

To some degree any medication you take will be present in your milk, but some medications are present in greater concentrations than others depending on their chemical makeup. Drugs that remain in the body for a long time should be avoided because your baby will not be able to excrete them as readily as shorter-acting medications.

Fortunately, there are steps you can take to minimize risks to your baby. Some medications are better suited to breast-feeding than others. The corticosteroid prednisolone appears to be safe. Likewise, most NSAIDs are considered safe because they are found in low concentrations in breast milk. Those NSAIDs that are short-acting such as ibuprofen are preferable to longer-acting NSAIDs.

If you have rheumatoid arthritis and want to breast-feed, you should avoid many DMARDs, including methotrexate, until you complete breast-feeding.

Arthritis and Sexuality

Problems with sexual relations are often ignored when living with arthritis. Fewer than one in five people with arthritis talk about this issue with their healthcare providers.

Fortunately, you can take steps to protect and maintain your sexuality—perhaps the same steps you are taking to protect your muscles and joints.

Sexuality is a complex phenomenon that involves the mind as well as the body, and desire as well as performance. As we get older our bodies change in many ways. Just as our muscles tighten and cartilage wears down, so, too, does our sexual response change. Sometimes it can take longer to become aroused and longer to reach climax.

If you are a woman who is past menopause and not taking estrogen replacement therapy, you may have trouble becoming lubricated, and the wall of your vagina may thin, which can make intercourse painful. If you are a man, you may have trouble achieving an erection because the arteries leading to your penis have narrowed so that blood flow is compromised. This can be the result of the natural aging process or because of diabetes or hypertension (which both affect circulation).

Both women and men are affected by medications they are taking. Blood pressure medicine, certain antidepressants, and certain cancer treatments can all have an effect on sexuality. Arthritis can also affect sexuality, and if you develop arthritis when you are older, it can exacerbate the effects of aging and any other health conditions you might have. The aching joints and weak muscles that characterize arthritis can interfere with your ability to express yourself sexually and to make love with your partner. Pain or joint damage in the back, shoulders, hips, and knees can prevent you from enjoying sex or wanting to initiate it. And the medications you are taking to treat your disease can also interfere with sexual functioning at times.

Not surprisingly, once you experience these physical problems, you may also feel anxious, nervous, or depressed, which can further subdue your sexual feelings.

What You Can Do to Help Yourself

What you do to help your heart and joints may also help your love life. All the advice previously given in this book about a good diet, regular exercise, and joint protection will help you restore your sexual functioning. Here is why:

Diet and exercise. Eating right and building and maintaining your muscles benefit you on many levels. Your energy level will increase, and you'll be better able to support your weight. More stamina and less pain can only help enhance your sex life.

The resistance exercises we've mentioned in earlier chapters are particularly helpful because they help maintain and build muscles that would otherwise deteriorate. If you are concerned about sexual functioning, concentrate on building the muscles in the back, shoulders, arms, and hips.

Protecting your joints. Another strategy is to take the strain off your arthritic joints while you are making love to your partner. If your back, knees, or hips are aching, change positions so that they are protected. Lying on your side or on your back may be easier than taking the upper position in the missionary position, for instance. Or use pillows to support your sore joints. Your healthcare provider may be able to provide advice, or with some communication and a little experimentation, you may be able to find alternate positions yourself.

Other helpful hints. The following tips have worked for other people with arthritis:

- Take a warm shower before you have sex to relax your muscles.
- Pick a time of day when you are feeling most rested and energetic. This may not be at the end of a long day!
- Take your pain medications so that they are still effective while you are having sex.
- Try alternatives to intercourse such as massage, which can also be pleasurable and intimate.

How Your Healthcare Provider May Help

Your healthcare provider and your physical therapist may both be able to provide advice and resources about sexuality. Don't be surprised if you feel embarrassed bringing this issue up. Many healthcare providers do as well. But we're all human, and sexuality is one of the things that many people consider essential for their well-being and happiness. It's worth discussing. Be prepared to be persistent. Your healthcare provider may not know how to help, and you may have to ask for a referral.

Arthritis medications. If sexual functioning is important to you, mention it to your healthcare provider when discussing medications. Some medications may dampen your sexual desire and response, while others will not. The only way to know for sure is to raise the issue.

Physical therapy. When you meet with your physical therapist to discuss how to improve mobility and reduce pain, you'll likely discuss a number of real-life situations such as work and home. If sexuality is a concern, discuss this as well. Your physical therapist may be able to suggest particular exercises or joint protection strategies that will help you enjoy sex as much as you did before you had arthritis.

Additional options. Your local pharmacy has a number of over-the-counter products to help you if you are having problems with sexual function. For women, vaginal lotions such as *K-Y* and *Replens* can offset the decrease in lubrication that is typical when you reach menopause or if you have Sjögren's syndrome (characterized by dry eyes and mouth). Or you can talk to your healthcare provider about estrogen replacement therapy or an estrogen cream or estrogen ring, which supply estrogen only to your vagina. Both men and women who are experiencing a decrease in desire can benefit from testosterone replacement therapy (sometimes available in a patch for the skin).

Several new prescription medications are available to assist with sexual functioning. Sildenafil *(Viagra)*, which works by improving blood flow to the genitals, increases sexual desire and performance for many people. It has been approved by the FDA for men and is currently under investigation for women. A number of similar products are now in various stages of development and will be marketed in the next few years.

Talk with your healthcare provider if you would like to use *Viagra* or a similar product to see if it is safe for you (especially if you are taking other medications, which could interact with it), and whether your healthcare provider has any cautions.

CHAPTER 13

The Miracles of Surgery

Jim had always been an athlete. He played football in college and took up racquetball in his forties and tennis in his fifties. But for the past two or three years he had trouble getting off the bench at the end of a game. And now it was so bad he could hardly walk. After trying medication and physical therapy, he was ready for something more. His healthcare provider suggested surgery.

CHANCES ARE you will not need surgery. Most people with arthritis are able to control their pain and other symptoms with the right combination of diet, exercise, medication, and complementary therapies. But there are times when surgery is the best option. It was once viewed as a treatment of last resort, but as we've learned more, that has changed.

Pain relief and diminished function are the most common reasons for surgery. If your arthritis has not responded to other treatments, and has become unbearable, and it is interfering with daily tasks, then your healthcare provider may recommend surgery. In some cases the results of surgery are so dramatic that you no longer have to take pain medications.

Sometimes surgery is performed to correct an underlying structural problem, such as hip dysplasia (where the bones are not properly aligned) in the hopes that it will prevent arthritis later on. Or if you already have arthritis and are unable to move a particular joint much, then surgery may be necessary to restore joint stability and mobility. At other times surgery can restore the look and function of deformed joints, such as those in your wrists and hands.

Surgery is most often performed on the weight-bearing joints, especially the hips and knees, but surgical options exist for all major joints.

Finding a Surgeon

Your healthcare provider should be able to refer you to a surgeon for further evaluation and treatment. If not, ask your healthcare provider how you can find a good orthopedic surgeon, a physician who specializes in operations on the bones, joints, and muscles. Some orthopedic surgeons subspecialize in particular joints.

When you visit the surgeon for the first time, he or she should be able to explain the type of operation that will be performed, how it should correct the problem, the risks and benefits of the procedure, how you should prepare for surgery, and what to expect as you recover. Ask as many questions as you want.

Because surgery is a big step, you may want to get a second opinion before proceeding. Once again, your healthcare provider may be able to provide a referral to another surgeon. Rheumatologists are also good sources of referrals because they often work closely with orthopedic surgeons. Or call the American Academy of Orthopedic Surgeons to find the name of other orthopedic surgeons in your area. (See appendix A for more information.)

Preparing for Surgery

Surgery is only performed when the benefits of the procedure outweigh the risks. And like any invasive treatment, surgery does carry risks—of infection, of aggravating some other condition such as heart disease or diabetes, or simply of not working as well as you'd hoped.

You can minimize the risks by taking care of yourself, using the tips provided in chapter 3. If you're too heavy, lose weight to decrease the pressure on your joints, heart, and lungs, and improve your chances of recovery.

If you have gum disease or any kind of bacterial infection, get it treated before you undergo surgery. Such infections can spread through your bloodstream, affecting the joint just operated on. And if you have diabetes, high blood pressure, or some other chronic condition not related to arthritis, talk to your healthcare provider about how to prepare for surgery.

If you are taking medications for your arthritis, check with your healthcare provider and your surgeon about the changes you should make in your regimen before surgery. Aspirin and NSAIDs, for instance, affect blood platelet function and may therefore increase bleeding. Your healthcare provider may recommend stopping all aspirin and NSAID use before your operation. If you are taking a DMARD such as methotrexate or etanercept (*Enbrel*), talk with your rheumatologist about stopping your medication prior to surgery.

If you are undergoing a type of surgery that will require blood transfusions, consider banking some of your own blood ahead of time. Although the blood supply in the United States is safe, banking your own blood eliminates even the small risks posed by transfusions. This may not be possible, however, if you have anemia.

If you have rheumatoid arthritis, you may have to take extra steps to prepare for surgery. As discussed in chapter 7, rheumatoid arthritis is an immune system disorder that can cause fatigue and anemia as well as joint pain. In the weeks before surgery, therefore, you should pay special attention to nutrition to avoid anemia. Work with your healthcare provider to get any inflamed joints under control since inflammation can slow your recovery. If you are receiving a corticosteroid such as prednisone, you may receive a high dose of corticosteroids intravenously on the day of surgery. And because your immune system may be suppressed by some of the medications you are taking, talk with your surgeon about infection control and wound healing.

What to Expect Before Your Operation

During your first meeting with your orthopedic surgeon, he or she will discuss the type of operation that is best for you and when it should be done. But before you actually go in for surgery, you'll also undergo a number of preoperative tests, including blood tests, a physical, and X rays if they have not already been taken. You may also answer detailed questions about such things as allergies to medications and past use of anesthesia or painkillers. If you have a history of problems with breathing or heart trouble, your surgeon may also order tests to evaluate heart and lung function.

A nurse or patient educator should give you pamphlets or other information about what to expect and how to prepare for surgery. (If not, ask!) It is important not to eat or drink anything after midnight on the day of your surgery. Anything in your stomach, even water, could be vomited and choke you when you receive anesthesia.

Anesthesia and Pain Relief

Before you undergo surgery, talk with your orthopedic surgeon about the type of anesthesia that will be used. He or she may recommend that you talk directly to your anesthesiologist. The following are the major types of anesthesia used.

General anesthesia. You will be unconscious during the operation. Your anesthesiologist will monitor your vital signs while providing you with drugs intravenously or will cover your nose and mouth with a mask so you can inhale the drugs.

Regional anesthesia. You will remain conscious during the operation, but an entire region of your body (such as from your waist down) will be numb. Regional anesthesia is frequently used during operations on the lower extremities, such as total knee replacements. It can be administered through an epidural or a spinal injection. In an epidural the anesthesiologist injects drugs through a thin plastic tube into the space that surrounds your spinal cord (the epidural space). A spinal injection goes directly into the spinal fluid. For both regional and local anesthesia, you may also be given a sedative to help you relax during the operation. Your view of the procedure may be blocked, although you will be aware of what is going on in the operating room.

Local anesthesia. You will remain conscious during the operation, but the part of your body that is being operated on will be numb. Local anesthesia is accomplished by injection to block sensations from particular nerves or by spray or ointment.

You may feel some discomfort when you first wake up from anesthesia and in the days that follow your surgery. For that reason your nurse will provide some type of pain medication almost immediately after you leave the operating room.

There are many options for pain relief in the hospital. You may receive pain medication intravenously, by injection, or in pill form. An increasingly popular method is something called "patient-controlled analgesia," or PCA, which is delivered through an IV line attached to a small pump that you can control to release pain medication as needed. When your pain subsides sufficiently, you will be provided with some type of pain pills that you can continue to take at home.

What to Expect After Surgery

If you have arthroscopic surgery, you may go home the same day because it is a minimally invasive procedure. Recovery is relatively fast.

If you have undergone a more invasive procedure, as in the case of a total joint replacement, you may require hospitalization and will be transferred to a general floor. Nurses will check your vital signs. They may ask you to move your fingers or toes. You may be asked to cough periodically or to breathe in deeply. This not only helps rid your body of anesthesia but also helps prevent pneumonia.

A side effect of some anesthesia is that you may have trouble urinating for a few days, and a catheter may be inserted to assist you. To prevent blood clots, which can sometimes develop after surgery, you may have special surgical stockings that encourage your blood to circulate or do simple flexing motions with your hands and feet. Your surgeon may also prescribe a blood-thinning agent such as warfarin (*Coumadin*), which you may need to take for six to twelve weeks after surgery. This is generally done to reduce the risk of blood clots following total knee and hip replacement. Because blood-thinning medications can interact with other drugs, it is important that your physician knows all medications you are currently taking.

You may be given iron supplements in the weeks following surgery, especially if you had more invasive surgery. The blood loss during surgery may lead to anemia, and iron supplements will help restore your blood count.

To reduce the risk of infection following a total joint replacement, you may be given a course of antibiotics both during and immediately after surgery. Your new joint is at increased risk of infection for as long as the replacement lasts. For that reason your surgeon may also recommend that you take antibiotics as a preventive measure whenever you undergo a procedure that can introduce infectious agents into your bloodstream—for example, extensive dental work (even if it takes place ten years after your total joint replacement).

Before leaving the hospital you will schedule a postoperative visit with your surgeon so that he or she can monitor your progress and determine how well you are healing. Don't be surprised if it takes you as long as six months to be completely back to normal, depending on the type of joint surgery. You may find that you don't have as much energy as you once did or that you seem to catch colds and other minor bugs more frequently. When you undergo surgery, many tissues have to heal. The best thing you can do for yourself is get enough rest, ease back into an exercise routine, and eat a nutritious diet. Your body needs all the help it can get to heal.

Physical Therapy

Don't be surprised if your surgeon and nurses have you up and moving sooner than you expect. Although bed rest and joint protection are important to your recovery, so are moving the affected joint and maintaining muscle tone throughout your body. Your physical therapist will undoubtedly be among your first visitors!

Initially, whatever joint has been operated on will be protected in some way. Your hand and arm may be placed in a protective splint to immobilize them. Your foot may be placed in an orthosis. The area may be covered with a surgical bandage until the incision heals sufficiently.

As soon as feasible, your physical therapist will ask you to do gentle range-of-motion exercises. You might wiggle your toes and flex your fingers, for instance. You might flex your knees and calves if your hip has been operated on. Following knee surgery, your leg may be placed in a device that provides continuous passive motion.

As swelling in the area decreases and your joint heals, you will begin strengthening exercises to build the muscles around the joints. The particular exercises you do will depend on the type of surgery you have had. If you had knee surgery, for instance, your physical therapist will ask you to concentrate on building your quadriceps muscles, located in your thigh, which provide support to your knee. See chapter 10 for details about joint-specific exercises.

Tips for Recovering at Home

Before you leave the hospital, your nurse or physical therapist will ask you about your home environment and suggest how you can make simple adaptations to better ensure your recovery. These may include the following:

- You may need to relearn how to sit down and get up from a chair or toilet to take the strain off your recovering joint.
- Remove any scatter rugs or anything you could trip on.
- You may have to be shown how to safely take a bath or shower; a shower seat or chair may be useful until you regain your strength and your joint heals.
- You'll have to learn how to get into bed and how to sleep so that your joint heals properly. For instance, if your hip was operated on, you may have to sleep with a pillow between your knees to prevent your hip from rotating inward.
- You may have to learn new techniques to dress yourself and to cook if your upper body (shoulders, elbows, hands) have been operated on.
- You may not be able to drive for a while.

Your physical therapist will also discuss ways to protect your joints at home and at work to enable them to continue healing properly.

Health Insurance and Money Issues

Surgery can be life changing, and it can affect your wallet as much as your joints. Before you decide on surgery, double-check your health insurance policy (or Medicaid or Medicare plan if you're eligible) to see which charges will be covered in full and which will not. In this era of managed care, coverage can change yearly, and you don't want to be surprised by a huge bill afterward. (That's the kind of pain no medication can help.)

Costs of surgery vary widely depending on the type of operation you undergo, the type of replacement parts and other materials that are used, the type of anesthesia that is used, and the type of medical professionals you have on your surgical team. Some insurance policies cover all professional services but only a portion of hospital costs. Others may require that you have your surgery in a particular hospital or network. Or your health insurance may cover only a certain number of days in a hospital. There may also be annual limits on the amount of reimbursement you can receive from your health plan (and surgery may put you over the limit if you've visited the doctor frequently).

This can be extremely confusing, but it's essential to know before you undergo surgery. Bring your health policy to your surgeon and ask about reimbursement questions. Some hospitals also have the equivalent of "financial aid" offices to help you sort out the details and your options.

Types of Surgery

A number of different surgical procedures are available to treat arthritis, ranging from repair to replacement of joints. The exact procedure your surgeon recommends will depend on your age, overall physical condition, and degree of damage in the affected joint. The types of surgery are as follows:

Arthroscopy. This minimally invasive surgery is often done on an outpatient basis, which reduces the time needed to recover. The surgeon makes a tiny incision and operates with the help of an arthroscope, a pen-sized instrument with a videoscope, attached to a monitor, in order to "see" inside the joint.

Bone fusion (**arthrodesis**). Your surgeon will bind two bones using pins, screws, or plates. As the bones heal, they bind together. Arthrodesis is effective at reducing pain and making the area more stable, but you will not be able to move the joint afterward.

Joint replacement (**arthroplasty**). Your surgeon will remove your damaged joint and replace it with artificial parts made of plastic or metal. Some replacement joints are cemented into place; others are textured so that your bone will grow around them, securing them. This procedure is reserved for severely damaged joints.

Soft tissue repair. As your joints are destroyed, they may also become deformed. Muscles, tendons, and ligaments can tear or actually separate from the bones. Your surgeon may repair the damage by tightening, loosening, or reattaching tendons, ligaments, and muscles.

Synovectomy. A synovial membrane surrounds each mobile joint and can become inflamed as a result of arthritis. In a synovectomy your surgeon removes part of the synovial membrane to reduce inflammation and pain.

Hand and Wrist

The bones and joints in our hands are relatively small, but their function is enormous. We get around during the day by using our hands as much as our feet. We may walk to the bus stop, but we use our hands to open the door so we can go outside in the first place. We may stand up to give a presentation, but chances are that we used our hands to prepare overheads, jot down notes for the talk, and collate and staple our handouts.

Small wonder, then, that hand surgery accounts for about one in four arthritis surgeries. If you have developed arthritis in your hands so severe that you can no longer open doors, dress or feed yourself, or make a living, then surgery may be your best option.

Hand surgery is challenging since bones, cartilage, muscles, tendons, and ligaments all come together in such relatively tight quarters. When a thumb joint is repaired, for instance, tendons may have to be replaced and ligaments attached.

In fact, the structures in your hand are as interdependent as the proverbial house of cards. One unhealthy joint can upset the delicate balance of muscles, tendons, ligaments, and bones, and more damage will result. For instance, if one joint in your hand develops arthritis, additional stress is placed on the adjacent joints when you begin to compensate for the one that is sore. Meanwhile, the muscles, tendons, and ligaments that provide support and structure may strain under the new pressure. In rheumatoid arthritis the area becomes inflamed, and the tendons may actually tear or rupture as well as the hand becomes deformed and fingers curl into unnatural positions. Fortunately, hand surgery offers several options to prevent or repair this type of damage.

Fusion (Arthrodesis)

Bone fusion is used most often in the wrist and seldom in the thumb or fingers. Partial fusion surgery enables your surgeon to stabilize and strengthen the wrist area without your having to lose complete flexibility. Both limited and total fusion will reduce pain and improve strength. The cost is lack of flexibility in your wrist.

Soft Tissue Repair

Tendon and ligament repair is another option, especially for the fingers and wrist. If you have rheumatoid arthritis, your tendons may tighten, loosen, or even tear away from the bone—all of which affect your ability to move your fingers and hand. In soft tissue repair your surgeon will realign bones and reattach tendons and ligaments. If the tendons are too badly damaged, replacement tendons taken from elsewhere in your body will be used to reconstruct the joint.

Joint Replacement (Arthroplasty)

Joint replacement is most often used in the hand to treat severe arthritis of the thumb and knuckles (the metacarpal joints). Rarely is joint replacement used for arthritis that affects other finger joints, such as in Heberden's or Bouchard's nodes. Joint replacement may also be done on the wrist, but this is not done as frequently as for the knee or hips.

Synovectomy

If rheumatoid arthritis has damaged your finger and wrist joints, your surgeon may recommend synovectomy to reduce pain and inflammation. Unfortunately, the symptoms may recur if the area becomes inflamed again.

Elbow

Your elbow exists mainly to move your hand to where you want it, and if you develop severe elbow arthritis, even the simplest movements, such as carrying a briefcase, may become impossible. Fortunately, if your arthritis does reach that point, you do have options.

Arthroscopy

This is used both to diagnose and to treat elbow arthritis. Your surgeon may use it to remove part of your elbow's synovial membrane or to smooth roughened cartilage and remove bone and cartilage bits that cause pain and aggravate the joint.

Synovectomy

This is one of the few surgeries recommended early rather than later in the course of rheumatoid arthritis. The goal is not only to reduce pain and inflammation but also to help prevent destruction of the elbow joint.

Total Joint Replacement (Arthroplasty)

In total elbow replacement your surgeon will replace the damaged portion of the joints with artificial parts. Some prostheses are hinged, others are not connected. This operation will reduce pain and increase function, often dramatically, but it is important not to overwork your new elbow. Because the elbow handles so much stress—by some estimates as much as three times your body weight when lifting heavy objects—implants can sometimes become dislocated or fail altogether.

Shoulder

Shoulder joints are the most mobile and in some ways the most useful of all the joints in the upper body. The shoulder is a ball-and-socket joint consisting of the humerus (the ball) and the glenoid (the socket). The joints attached to the clavicle and shoulder blades also contribute to movement.

Arthritis in your shoulder also affects the ability to move your elbow and hands. Some people with severe shoulder arthritis are not able to lift a bowl of soup. Surgery of the shoulder therefore aims not only at reducing pain but at restoring function.

The shoulder presents a number of challenges when it comes to surgery. The joint is mobile not only because of its intricate structure but also because fourteen muscles act upon the humerus, scapula, and clavicle. Your surgeon has to pay close attention to the muscles and tendons holding the joint in place as well as to the joint itself. Physical therapy becomes especially important for recovery.

Arthroscopy

This procedure allows a better look inside the shoulder to determine the extent of the damage. Arthroscopy may be used to remove small amounts of the synovial membrane or bits of cartilage and bone to restore the joint to a healthier state.

Total Joint Replacement (Arthroplasty)

The surgeon replaces both the humerus and glenoid in the shoulder. This operation relieves pain and improves function. It is also very successful when done early, before you have suffered severe joint damage. Because mobility in the shoulder depends as much on muscles as on the actual joint structure, the extent of function you recover in your shoulder will depend to a large degree on how successful your surgeon is at repairing the muscles and other soft tissues as well as the shoulder joint itself.

Hip

Total hip replacement is the most common type of surgery for arthritis. Small wonder. Our hips bear much of our weight and are responsible for much of our ability to walk and move around. You may be a candidate for surgery if you are experiencing constant pain in your buttocks, hips, and/or groin, particularly if it is bad enough to wake you at night or you have started to limp.

Your hips, like your shoulders, are ball-and-socket joints. And like your shoulders, they withstand enormous stress. Just walking up the stairs, which requires that you put all your weight first on one leg and then the other, places four times your body's weight on your hips. The goals of hip surgery are to reduce the pressure on the joint, thereby decreasing pain and the chance of further joint damage, and to restore function.

Total Hip Replacement (Arthroplasty)

In this surgery the surgeon replaces the ball-and-socket joint with an artificial one (see below). Total hip replacement is one of the success stories of orthopedic surgery. It was first introduced in the 1960s. Since then, improvements in materials available to make artificial joints, as well as better techniques, have combined so that the replacement joints last longer. A hip replacement should last for ten to twenty years, and perhaps longer.

Some of the artificial joints are cemented into place; others are designed so that your bone grows into the artificial joint, securing it in place. Although your surgeon will select the type of prosthesis you receive based on your age, hip damage, and activity level, generally the joints that do not require cement are used in people younger than fifty. Hybrid hip implants consist of a cemented thighbone (femur) and uncemented hip socket (acetabulum). This design is used frequently and is quite effective.

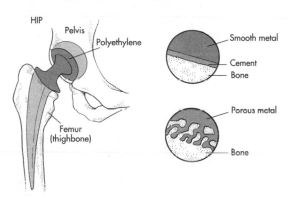

Artificial Hip Joint

Artificial joints have metal shafts that are inserted into bone and anchored. At weight-bearing points, slick high-density polyethylene is used to reduce friction, as cartilage does in natural joints.

Cement is used to fasten the artificial joint to the bone in many joint-replacement operations.

Cementless implants have a porous surface that bone tissue grows into, holding the prosthesis in place.

No matter what type of artificial joint is used, the surgeon will remove the top of the thighbone and bore a hole into it. This will hold the replacement for the ball part of the joint. Then the surgeon reshapes the socket part of the hip, located in the pelvic bone. The artificial joint then fits neatly into the space, creating a new joint.

Once you recover from surgery, the results may astound you. You may no longer be in pain, and you may find you are able to do activities you gave up long ago. Recovery takes time, however; it could be two or three months before you are back to normal. But when you do recover, you may feel ten years younger.

Knee

Along with our hips, our knees bear the brunt of much of our weight and our activities. It's not uncommon for knees to withstand three to six times our weight, especially if we are running or doing high-impact aerobics. (As discussed in chapter 2, muscles and ligaments provide support to the knee, with cartilage providing a secondary shock absorber.) Not surprisingly, then, knee surgery is among the most commonly performed for arthritis.

Arthroscopy

Sometimes arthroscopy is used to diagnose a problem that cannot be detected through X ray or MRI imaging of the area. At other times arthroscopy is used to correct damage to knee cartilage, ligaments, or joint (see Arthroscopic Knee Surgery on page 319). You can recover from arthroscopy quickly. Generally you go home the day of the operation and resume normal activities within a month.

Total Joint Replacement (Arthroplasty)

The results of this operation can be dramatic in terms of reduced pain and increased mobility. In total joint replacement your surgeon removes the diseased and damaged portions of the knee and replaces them with artificial materials—usually made of polyethylene. (See Artificial Knee Joint on page 319.)

Arthroscopic Knee Surgery

In arthroscopic knee surgery, two small incisions are made to create portals for the arthroscope and irrigator, which infuses sterile fluid into the joint to distend it. Other incisions are made to accommodate surgical instruments that may be needed to cut, shave, remove particles, or repair tissue.

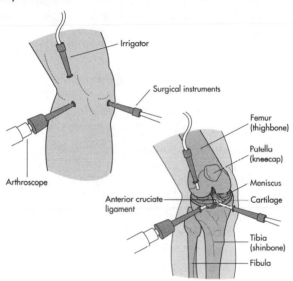

Artificial Knee Joint

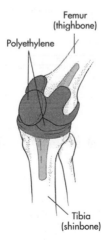

You will remain in the hospital for four or five days following the operation. Within three to six months you should be back to normal.

Knee replacements should last from ten to fifteen (and sometimes even twenty) years depending on weight and activity level. No matter how well done the surgery, artificial knees may loosen up with time. The more you can avoid contact and high-impact activities, the better.

Foot and Ankle

Your foot may be small relative to the rest of your body, but it has the strength of a giant. If you are 150 pounds and walk for a mile, you have placed about 63 tons of cumulative weight on each foot! Fortunately, your foot and ankle are designed to withstand and redistribute this pressure. Sometimes this engineering marvel breaks down, however, and you develop arthritis in your foot. Or you may develop arthritis in your foot as a result of a misalignment somewhere else that places more pressure on an otherwise healthy structure. If the disease progresses, you may need surgery.

Foot surgery may be appropriate for your ankle, forefoot, or hindfoot and can range from a relatively simple repair of a particular joint to a total ankle replacement. It is rare for an entire portion of the foot to be replaced.

Postoperative recovery time depends on the operation used and the joint or joints involved. Sometimes a special postoperative shoe is needed to keep the foot immobile for weeks or even months or the foot is taped or placed in a cast so it can heal.

Procedures Under Investigation

Several procedures are under investigation and may provide additional surgical options in the future. These include bone and cartilage transplants as well as methods to actually grow new tissue.

Questions for Your Surgeon

1. What kind of operation do you recommend and why?
2. What experience do you have with this type of surgery? Could you give me the name of another patient who has undergone this operation?
3. What other alternatives do I have besides surgery?
4. What type of results should I expect (such as pain relief, increased mobility, etc.)?
5. What should I do to prepare for surgery? Should I make any change in my medications?
6. What type of anesthesia will be used? What are the benefits? What are the possible complications?
7. How long will I stay in the hospital?
8. How long will it take for me to recover from the operation?
9. Will I need to wear a cast or splint of some type after surgery? Will I need to walk on crutches or use a cane?
10. Will I have to keep the joint immobile? How long?
11. Are there adaptations I should make to my home in order to recover better?
12. Will I need help getting dressed and eating?
13. Will I have to enter a rehabilitation facility or nursing home, or can I go directly home?
14. What other restrictions will be placed on my activities following surgery? When can I drive? Return to work? Do housework? Have sex?
15. What type of physical therapy may be necessary? Can you refer me to a physical therapist?
16. What type of supplies should I buy ahead of time? What supplies will be provided to me?
17. How many follow-up visits will be required? Are they included in the fee?
18. Will surgery have to be performed again in the future?

In cartilage transplantation, healthy chrondrocytes (a component of cartilage) are removed from the joint and cultured in a laboratory so that they multiply. The cultured cells are then reinjected into the joint where cartilage has eroded. The hope is that these transplanted cells will grow into new cartilage, replacing the damaged tissue.

So far this procedure has had promising results. It appears to work best when used to repair small areas of damage rather than large-scale joint destruction. The FDA has approved it for knee damage due to injury but not for arthritis. The procedure remains under investigation.

Similarly, bone cells have been transplanted into damaged bone to see if new bone will form and repair the area. Early results have been mixed, and further investigation is needed before this practice can become mainstream.

Further on the horizon are methods that may actually grow new bone and cartilage from stem cells (which give rise to the more specialized cells that form our organs and the rest of our bodies). This tissue-engineering approach might also work for damaged tendons and ligaments. This research is in the earliest phases but provides a whole new approach to the problem of arthritis.

CHAPTER 14

Putting It All Together

WE HOPE this book has been informative. In order to assist you in weaving the various strands of information together so that you can craft your own arthritis management plan, we offer here typical situations in the hope that you find one close to your own.

Case Study #1: Concerned About the Future

Pam was never concerned about arthritis until she banged her knee hard one day. For two days she hobbled around, stiff and uncomfortable. The problem went away, but Pam was shaken. She was in decent physical shape at forty-two because she dieted, not because she excrcised. (Who had time, between working full time and juggling the kids' schedules?) But limping around for a few days was enough to make her reconsider her priorities. Maybe she was too busy taking care of everyone else's needs—satisfying her kids and her boss, juggling travel schedules with her husband—and wasn't paying enough attention to her own. She certainly didn't want to end up like her aunt Edna who was using a walker to get around because of advanced osteoarthritis of the knee.

"How do I protect myself?" wondered Pam.

Putting Together a Prevention Plan

Banging your knee hard provides some insight into the pain and limited mobility that arthritis might bring. Consider it a wake-up call. To reduce the risk of arthritis, take steps to improve overall health and fitness such as:

Start exercising. Primary support to your joints is provided by the muscles, which help to brace the area and absorb the shock of impact. See chapter 3 for tips on exercising.

Watch your diet. Calcium and vitamin D supplements reduce the risk of developing osteoporosis later on. A well-balanced diet promotes all-around good health. See chapter 2.

Practice good work habits. As we age, our muscles tighten and become less flexible. At twenty-two we can twist sideways to retrieve a file while cradling the phone receiver between ear and shoulder, but at forty-two we're liable to injure ourselves. See chapter 10 for tips on how to protect joints.

Reduce stress. Sometimes we walk into things when we are feeling tired or preoccupied. To reduce stress, try some of the complementary therapies discussed in chapter 11, such as meditation and visualization, or have some herbal tea.

Buy comfortable shoes. Women are more likely than men to develop osteoarthritis of the knees. Some experts think that high heels, which redistribute weight so that more pressure is placed on the knees, may explain why. To be safe, wear shoes with low heels and wide toe areas.

Case Study #2: Preventing Further Damage

Joe had been a carpenter for years, pounding nails into two-by-fours and hauling building supplies up and down ladders. He worked in all kinds of weather, often with the foreman chiding him about finishing the project on time. His wife, Bobbie, was a data processor. Like Joe, she was under pressure to work at a fast pace. She seldom got up from her chair when she was at work so that she wouldn't lag behind the others.

Recently, Joe and Bobbie joked about getting old. She was dropping things, such as her car keys and even a bottle of milk. He had trouble pushing the lawn mower on Saturdays, his thumbs were so sore. Their healthcare provider told Joe he had a mild case of osteoarthritis in his thumbs. Bobbie had carpal tunnel syndrome and the beginnings of osteoarthritis in her hands. Now what?

Managing Mild Osteoarthritis

Managing mild pain and loss of function from osteoarthritis requires a multiprong approach:

Rest and protect the injured joints. Joints can take a lot of pressure (see chapter 2), but repeated stress on any joint, especially if it is high impact, may cause damage. To take a load off (literally), try using thumb and wrist splints (see chapter 10) and take breaks to stand and stretch occasionally.

Strengthen muscles. If a joint is sore, it's not getting enough support. Finger, hand, and wrist exercises are discussed in chapter 10.

Control pain. Mild to moderate pain can be alleviated using over-the-counter products available at any pharmacy. Try acetaminophen (found in *aspirin-free Excedrin* and *Tylenol*) first, and if that doesn't work, try an NSAID such as ibuprofen *(Advil)* or naproxen *(Aleve).*

Exercise. To help reduce pain in any affected joint and to prevent arthritis from developing in other joints, there are three major types of exercise (see chapter 3). Maintain flexibility by trying tai chi or yoga, described in chapter 12.

Apply heat or cold. These can be applied to sore joints or used to prepare for exercise. See chapter 10 for more details.

Try complementary therapies. Glucosamine and chondroitin sulfate may be of help. For more information, see chapter 11.

Case Study #3: Revising the Game Plan

Valerie was tired of being so dependent on medication. She took one type of pill for her high blood pressure, another for her depression, and still another for the osteoarthritis in her left knee. Sometimes she took five or six pills a day when the pain was bad. What's more, her insurance plan balked at paying for one of the newer drugs being advertised, and she did not have enough money to pay for it herself. Because she felt sore, she wasn't exercising the way her healthcare provider suggested. Now she was gaining weight, and that made her feel even worse. There had to be a better way.

Multiple Strategies to Control Pain

When pain from osteoarthritis is moderate, or even severe, then it may seem absurd to rely on anything but medication to control it. Yet there are a number of different alternatives that may prove valuable. And exercise and diet should always be part of the mix.

Have a massage. Dealing with several conditions at once—high blood pressure, depression, osteoarthritis—can be difficult. Take time out and get a massage. This improves mood and loosens muscles, which can reduce pain. See chapter 11.

Try acupuncture. A number of studies have reported that acupuncture can significantly reduce pain caused by osteoarthritis—without medication. Check to see if your health insurance plan will cover it. (See chapter 11.)

Lose weight. There is no way around it: The heavier you are, the more pressure you are placing on your joints. See chapter 3 about a good diet. If you are intimidated by the thought of exercising, start with something gentle and noncompetitive. See more about movement therapies in chapter 12.

Ask about assistive devices. Splints, braces, and orthotic devices allow tired, sore joints to rest and will help reduce pain. See chapter 10.

Switch medications. When pain persists even after trying different strategies, it may be time to switch to another medication. Drugs work differently from one person to the next, or you may need a different dose. Talk with your healthcare provider and see chapter 5 for a description of the various medications available.

Case Study #4: Fighting Back

When Denise learned she had rheumatoid arthritis, her first reaction was shock, followed quickly by anger. How could she have a chronic and potentially debilitating disease at the age of thirty-four? She didn't stay angry long. Shortly after her diagnosis, Denise and her rheumatologist developed an aggressive treatment plan that made her feel more in the driver's seat.

Medication. Rheumatoid arthritis is best treated early and aggressively. Some of the most effective relief can be found in the early administration of a disease-modifying anti-rheumatic drug (DMARD) such as methotrexate. (See chapter 7 for more information about DMARDs and chapter 5 for information about pain relief.)

Join a support group. It is difficult to learn that you have a chronic disease. One of the best ways to educate yourself quickly about rheumatoid arthritis and receive emotional support from people who understand what you are going through is to join a support group. Contact the Arthritis Foundation for a support group in your area. (See a list of helpful organizations in appendix A.)

Surf the Web for information. The Internet and the World Wide Web are creating virtual communities for people with arthritis. See the list of Web sites in appendix A and explore a few. (Some include tips on coping and where to find helpful products.) One word of caution: Anyone can post information on the Web, and much of it is erroneous. Look for sites hosted by the federal government or by credible institutions.

Reconsider priorities. Like any autoimmune disease, rheumatoid arthritis may cause fatigue as well as other symptoms. If you are in a fast-paced job, work long hours, and seldom take breaks, this may be the time to reconsider your priorities. You will need to rest regularly throughout the day and keep stress to a minimum so that you have the energy to cope with symptoms. See chapter 12 for more information.

Try complementary therapies. Evening primrose oil and fish oil supplements reduce some of the signs of inflammation, and many people with rheumatoid arthritis find them helpful when used in conjunction with medications like DMARDs. See chapter 11 for more information. (Also take a look at some of the relaxation techniques discussed.)

Case Study #5: Trying Something New

For several years Jane took high doses of non-steroidal anti-inflammatory drugs (NSAIDs) for her rheumatoid arthritis, and then she ended up in the hospital with an ulcer. Fortunately, it healed. But she was worried it would recur. She was also concerned that the constant inflammation in her hands would destroy them; certainly they were all but useless when she had flares. Jane didn't want to become disabled, but she was beginning to wonder how much longer she could keep working.

Taking Advantage of Medical Advances

In the past five years there has been a surge in the development of drugs for the treatment of rheumatoid arthritis. There have also been advances in understanding nontraditional approaches to managing this disease. If you have not responded well to traditional medications, it may be time to try something new.

COX-2 inhibitors. If you have had an ulcer or are at increased risk of gastrointestinal bleeding, then ask your rheumatologist about the new COX-2 inhibitors *(Celebrex* and *Vioxx).* These provide the same pain and inflammation relief as NSAIDs but cause fewer ulcers.

Biological response modifiers and newer DMARDs. One of the most exciting developments in the past few years has been the discovery of drugs that target specific immune system cells that mistakenly attack joints. Two biological response modifiers, etanercept *(Enbrel)* and infliximab *(Remicade),* and the new drug leflunomide *(Arava)* interfere with the disease process itself. These medications can also be combined with the more traditional disease-modifying anti-rheumatic drugs (DMARDs). See chapter 7 for more information.

Physical therapy. Our appreciation of the ways that physical therapy can help preserve joint function and reduce pain has also increased in the past five to ten years. If you are taking high-dose medications for rheumatoid arthritis, you should visit a physical therapist to see if there are other ways to find relief for the pain and inflammation. He or she can provide advice about splints, braces, and orthotic devices that can ease the strain on joints and advice about exercises to retain as much function as possible. See chapter 10.

Oil your joints. Recently, we learned that omega-3 fatty acids, found in fish such as mackerel and salmon, and in supplements, helps reduce pain and inflammation. Consuming more of this type of oil per week is a good complement to your medications and physical therapy. See chapter 11 for more information.

Journal writing. One of the more intriguing studies to come along recently reported that people with rheumatoid arthritis who write about their stressful experiences suffer fewer symptoms. It doesn't take long—only twenty minutes a day—to enjoy the benefits. See chapter 11 for more information.

Organizations That Can Provide More Information

Best places to begin:

American College of Rheumatology
1800 Century Place, Suite 250
Atlanta, GA 30345
404-633-3777
Web site: www.rheumatology.org

The Arthritis Foundation
1330 West Peachtree Street
Atlanta, GA 30309
404-872-7100
Toll free: 800-283-7800
Web site: www.arthritis.org

For additional information about specific subjects:

American Academy of Medical
Acupuncture
5820 Wilshire Boulevard, Suite 500
Los Angeles, CA 90036
323-937-5514
Toll free: 800-521-2262
Web site:
www.medicalacupuncture.org

American Academy of
Orthopaedic Surgeons
6300 North River Road
Rosemont, IL 60018
847-823-7186 (main line)
Toll free: 800-346-2267 (main line)
Toll free: 800-824-2663 (for a list
of free publications)
Web site: www.aaos.org

American Academy of Pain
Management
13947 Mono Way #A
Sonora, CA 95370
209-533-9744
Web site: www.aapainmanage.org

The American Botanical Council
P.O. Box 144345
Austin, TX 78714
512-926-4900
Web site: www.herbalgram.org

American Chronic Pain Association
P.O. Box 850
Rocklin, CA 95677
916-632-0922
Web site: www.theacpa.org

American Dietetic Association
216 West Jackson Boulevard
Chicago, IL 60606
312-899-0040
Web site: www.eatright.org

The American Juvenile Arthritis
Organization
A council of The Arthritis Foundation
1330 West Peachtree Street
Atlanta, GA 30309
404-965-7538
Toll free: 800-283-7800
Web site: www.arthritis.org

American Pain Society
4700 West Lake Avenue
Glenview, IL 60025-1485
847-375-4715
Web site: www.ampainsoc.org

American Podiatric Medical
  Association
9312 Old Georgetown Road
Bethesda, MD 20814
301-571-9200
Toll free: 800-275-2762
Web site: www.apma.org

The Food and Drug Administration
Rockville, MD 20857
Toll free: 888-INFO-FDA
  (888-463-6332)
Web site: www.fda.org

Lyme Disease Foundation
1 Financial Plaza
Hartford, CT 06103
860-525-2000
Web site: www.lyme.org

The National Center for
  Complementary Medicine,
  National Institutes of Health
  (NCCAM) Clearinghouse
P.O. Box 8218
Silver Spring, MD 20907
Toll free: 888-644-6226
Web site: nccam.nih.gov

National Institute of Arthritis &
  Musculo-Skeletal and Skin Diseases
Information Clearinghouse
National Institutes of Health
1 AMS Circle
Bethesda, MD 20892
301-495-4484
Toll free: 877-226-4267
Web site: www.nih.gov/niams

Spondylitis Association of America
14827 Ventura Boulevard, Suite 222
Sherman Oaks, CA 91403
Toll free: 800-777-8189
Web site: www.spondylitis.org

For Further Reading
or More Information

To order books, newsletters, and other materials from the Arthritis Foundation, call 800-207-8633 toll free. Many of the materials listed here (regardless of publisher) are also available at your local bookstore or through online services such as www.amazon.com or www.bn.com. Prices vary.

Books

The Arthritis Foundation's Guide to Alternative Therapies by Judith Horstman. Atlanta: Arthritis Foundation, 1999.

The Arthritis Helpbook: A Tested Self-Management Program for Coping with Arthritis and Fibromyalgia by Kate Lorig, R.N., Dr.Ph. and James F. Fries, M.D. Cambridge, Mass.: Perseus Books, 2000.

Arthritis 101: Questions You Have, Answers You Need. Atlanta: Arthritis Foundation, 1997.

Beyond Chaos: One Man's Journey Alongside His Chronically Ill Wife by Gregg Piburn. Atlanta: Arthritis Foundation, 1999.

Celebrate Life: New Attitudes for Living with Chronic Illness. Atlanta: Arthritis Foundation, 1999.

Help Yourself: Recipes and Resources from the Arthritis Foundation. Atlanta: Arthritis Foundation.

Making Sense of Fibromyalgia. Atlanta: Arthritis Foundation.

The People's Pharmacy Guide to Home and Herbal Remedies by Joe Graedon and Teresa Graedon, Ph.D. New York: St. Martin's Press, 1999.

Raising a Child with Arthritis: A Parent's Guide. Atlanta: Arthritis Foundation, 1998.

Rheumatic Disease Clinics of North America. Complementary and Alternative Therapies for Rheumatic Diseases, vols 1 and 2 (Feb. 2000), edited by Richard S. Panush, M.D. Philadelphia: WB Saunders Company, 1999, 2000.

250 Tips for Making Life with Arthritis Easier. Atlanta: Arthritis Foundation.

Walk with Ease: Your Guide to Walking for Better Health, Improved Fitness and Less Pain. Atlanta: Arthritis Foundation, 1999.

Your Personal Guide to Living Well with Fibromyalgia. Atlanta: Arthritis Foundation.

Magazines and Newsletters

Arthritis Today
The Arthritis Foundation
1330 West Peachtree Street
Atlanta, GA 30309
Toll free: 800-933-0032

Fibromyalgia Health Newsletter
The Arthritis Foundation
1330 West Peachtree Street
Atlanta, GA 30309
Toll free: 877-755-0343

Kids Get Arthritis Too
American Juvenile Arthritis Organization
P.O. Box 921907
Norcross, GA 30010
Toll free: 800-268-6942

Web Sites

In addition to the Web sites listed in appendix A you may want to visit the following sites. Be aware that anything that ends in .gov is a government-sponsored site and .edu is a college or university-based site. We have not included any commercial sites (those that end in .com) because the information they contain may not have been evaluated by a medical expert and there may be a profit motive guiding the information presented.

Generally speaking, the government sites are the most trustworthy because the medical information has been verified by a medical expert and there is no commercial interest in the information being shared. No Web site can substitute for your own healthcare provider's advice.

The Harvard Medical School update site (which provides updates on the material presented in this book)
www.health.harvard.edu

The Centers for Disease Control
www.cdc.gov

Healthfinder, sponsored by the U.S. Department of Health and Human Services
www.healthfinder.gov

New York Online Access to Health offers materials in Spanish and English
www.noah.cuny.edu

Illustrations and Tables Credits

Illustrations on the following pages are copyright © Harriet Greenfield, West Newton, Mass.: 25, 30, 45, 47, 49, 167, 317, and 319.

Illustrations on the following pages are copyright © Hilda Muinos, MS, CMI, at www.muinosmedicalvisuals.com: 114, 120, 121, 225, 226, 227, 228, 229, 230, 231, 232, 233, 236, 237, 238, 239, 241, 288, 289, 291, 292, and 293.

Hilda Muinos's illustration of Heberden's and Bouchard's Nodes on page 114 is adapted from Susan Keller's illustration in Karen J. Carlson, Stephanie A. Eisenstat, and Terra Ziporyn, *The Harvard Guide to Women's Health* (Cambridge: Harvard University Press, 1996), p. 442.

Hilda Muinos's illustrations, "Isometric Exercise" (page 120) and "Isotonic Exercise" (page 121), are adapted from "Exercise and Your Arthritis," The Arthritis Foundation, Atlanta, Ga., pp. 7–8. Copyright © 1999. Used by permission of The Arthritis Foundation, 1330 West Peachtree Street, Atlanta, GA 30309. For more information, please call The Arthritis Foundation's Information Line at 800-283-7800 or log on to www.arthritis.org.

Hilda Muinos's illustrations on pages 225–233, 236, and 241 are adapted from illustrations by Jerry O'Brien in Margaret Hills and Janet Horwood, *Exercise and Arthritis: A Guide to Pain-Free Movement* (Allentown Penn.: People's Medical Society, 1997), pp. 42, 44, 46–48, 52–55, and 74–78.

Hilda Muinos's illustrations on pages 237–239 are adapted from a Rehabilitation Services handout, courtesy of Brigham and Women's Hospital, Boston, Mass.

Hilda Muinos's illustrations on pages 288 and 289 are adapted from Sophia Delza's illustrations in Sophia Delza, *T'ai Chi Ch'üan: Body and Mind in Harmony* (North Canton, Ohio: Good News Edition in arrangement with David McKay Co., Inc., 1961), p. 65.

Hilda Muinos's illustrations on pages 291–293 are adapted from Evelyn England and Herbert Ascherman Jr.'s photographs in Alice Christensen, *The*

Index